41 Self-Discipline Tips
for Slackers, Avoiders, & Couch Potatoes

By Peter Hollins,
Author and Researcher at
petehollins.com

Table of Contents

CHAPTER 1: GETTING STARTED — 7

- SET SMALL GOALS FIRST — 7
- START ON A MONDAY — 10
- NEVER SKIP TWO DAYS IN A ROW — 14
- MONITOR YOUR PROGRESS — 17
- PUT YOUR GOALS WHERE YOU CAN SEE THEM — 20
- VISUALIZE YOUR OUTCOME — 23

CHAPTER 2: FOCUS ON HABITS — 31

- REPLACE OLD HABITS — 31
- EAT WELL, EAT REGULARLY — 35
- EXERCISE BODY... AND MIND — 40
- FINE TUNE YOUR MORNINGS — 43
- STICK TO A SCHEDULE — 47
- MAKE ROOM FOR BREAKS, TREATS, AND REWARDS — 51

CHAPTER 3: GET RIGHT IN YOUR BODY, MIND AND SOUL — 57

- REMOVE TEMPTATIONS — 57
- DON'T WAIT FOR IT TO "FEEL RIGHT" — 61
- FOCUS ON THE POSITIVE — 64
- MIND YOUR MOOD — 68
- LOWER OTHER LIFE STRESSORS — 72
- THE EMOTIONAL EATING CYCLE (AND HOW TO APPLY IT TO OTHER SITUATIONS) — 75
- SIP SOME LEMONADE! — 79

CHAPTER 4: THE ATTITUDE OF SUCCESS — 85

- STOP CALLING LAZINESS PRODUCTIVITY — 85

GET FRIENDS TO HOLD YOU ACCOUNTABLE	89
DETERMINE WHAT YOU CAN CONTROL	92
TAKE OWNERSHIP AND RESPONSIBILITY	96
PRACTICE GRATITUDE	99
BELIEVE IN WILLPOWER	103

CHAPTER 5: STAY MINDFUL — 109

MEDITATE TO ACTIVATE	109
KEEP CALM, KEEP MINDFUL	113
DROP THE EGO	116
KNOW THE DIFFERENCE BETWEEN SUFFERING AND PAIN	120
GET ACQUAINTED WITH YOUR WEAKNESSES	124

CHAPTER 6: GET ORGANIZED WITH YOUR TIME — 131

PUT THE BIG ROCKS IN FIRST	131
TIME MANAGEMENT ACCORDING TO YOUR UNIQUE RHYTHMS	135
THE POWER OF A COUNTDOWN	138
AVOID PROCRASTINATION—METHODS THAT WORK	141
CUT YOUR TO-DO LIST IN HALF	145
SEEK PATTERNS—AND CHANGE THEM	149

CHAPTER 7: WORKING WITH GOALS AND VISIONS — 155

LET VISON POWER YOUR DECISION	155
BE DECISIVE AND COMMITTED	159
GOALS: IDENTIFY THEM AND WRITE THEM DOWN	163
WHEN IN DOUBT, WRITE IT OUT	167
GET COMFORTABLE WITH UNCOMFORTABLE	171

SUMMARY GUIDE — 177

Chapter 1: Getting Started

Set small goals first

How do you eat an entire elephant? One bite at a time!

Corny jokes aside, i<u>t's *far easier to be disciplined about small things to start with and build momentum from there*</u>. Change is hard, and our brains are wired to return to what feels comfortable and predictable. That's why big changes can be so hard, and why we can often get overwhelmed staring at the big picture and seeing how far we have to go. But if you start slow, you can build momentum without getting overwhelmed.

If you want to start walking thirty minutes a day, five days a week, start with just five minutes a day. If you feel like continuing after five minutes, go for it! But all you have to focus on when you start is that crucial first step. That's all.

If you want to start eating better, identify just one change you can make in your diet. Keep that going for a while, then see where you are and what step to take next later. Often, when our mind thinks something is going to be easy, there's not much resistance to just starting. And then, once we start, we can immediately start to feel that sense of achievement, movement, and hope—and that allows us to begin to build momentum to keep going. The longer you stay in prep mode without starting, however, and the longer you contemplate the huge mountain ahead of you that you have to climb, the more immobilized you'll feel.

Try not to psych yourself out by setting the bar too high. Confidence should be built by setting and achieving a small goal before going for a bigger one. After all, what feels better, knowing you have a big project ahead of you, or knowing that you are *already* on the path and doing what you need to do? Be patient with yourself and try not to get frustrated with the process. Accomplishing those small goals first can give you the motivation and inspiration to take the next step. And the next!

It's easy to get caught up in the excitement of a big goal and forget that those big goals are really just a collection of lots and lots of little goals. And all you are really responsible for at any one time is a *single* one of those actions. Once you meet one goal, promise yourself you will look again and set the next one. But before then, your main job is just to get the current step completed. A lot of people believe that if they cannot summon the energy, money, time, or willpower to achieve the entire massive goal all at once, then they can't start and might as well not bother. But that's not true! You only need enough to do the very first step. Then bank that progress and look at the next step.

How to Use This in Your Life Immediately

Think about a goal in your life right now that has felt a little intimidating or overwhelming. Choose something that you have not felt confident or energetic enough to tackle. Look at this big action and break it down into as many tiny actions as you can. For example, if you wanted to write your one-hundred-thousand-word novel, well, that's just a question of writing one word one hundred thousand times over. Really! Set yourself the goal of writing one thousand words at a time. If that seems intimidating still, drop it to five hundred or one hundred. Choose the baby step that makes you think, "Oh, actually that's not such a big deal. I think I can do that." Then do that. Think *small*.

Start on a Monday

Human beings love a fresh start. It's seemingly in our DNA. Beginning any new project on the right day give you the opportunity to start over anew, and promotes self-improvement, motivation, and self-discipline. The most significant dates turn out to be, in this order: the first day of the year, the first day after a national holiday, and Monday, the first day of the week.

Monday gives us more motivation than other days of the week because it signals a new beginning. It works even better if the day has personal significance for you, such as a birthday, a holiday, or the start of a new job. Whatever it is, there is great power in harnessing the energy and enthusiasm that comes with a new leaf and a chance to start over again, no matter how small.

I know what you're thinking: you *hate* Mondays. You hate them so much sometimes that you start dreading them on Friday already, right? But you can transform this attitude into one where you're genuinely excited to begin again. Research in the journal *Psychological Science* has shown that people are actually more likely to follow through with new projects begun on a Monday. It's as though observing the start of the week gives you an extra boost, cements the new start in your mind, and tells your unconscious mind, "This is it—the start of something different."

It's a temporal landmark that allows you to wipe the slate clean, forget about where you've been, and turn your full enthusiasm to the week ahead and its goals. It's not so much that the week is new, but that *you* get to be a new person and make a clean break from any failures or missed opportunities of the past. Productivity gurus may say that the best time to start a new goal is this very instant, but there's something about the ceremony and markedness of a Monday that may in fact be more powerful.

How to Use This in Your Life Immediately

This tip is not free license to procrastinate all your work until next Monday! *How* you start on a Monday matters, too. It's worth saying that Monday is great, but you can also choose some other significant day—for example, if you have for years started your weekday on a Wednesday, then that may be more meaningful for you. If it's your birthday coming up in a few days, plan to start something new then, and signal to your unconscious mind that something new and fresh and exciting has begun. Here's how to go ahead with a Monday start date:

- Make a list and be prepared. On Sunday night (or better yet, Friday afternoon) make a plan for exactly what you're going to do come Monday morning. Don't "ease into it"—just start, and start with the big, important things first. Think about the most important first step and

knock that off the list as soon as possible so you can capitalize on that momentum and get yourself feeling excited and accomplished as soon as possible.
- Don't just plan the actions that relate to your goal directly. Also, plan the outfit you're going to wear that day (choose something clean, appropriate, and well-fitting that makes you feel like a million bucks) and make sure you have a breakfast plan lined up. Schedule your first cup of coffee for when you've already been up for one or two hours, for maximum efficiency.
- Supercharge your fresh start with fresh everything—fling open a window and fill your lungs with the air of a new day, open a fresh bar of soap, or wear a new pair of socks, and expose yourself to the new morning sun as soon as you wake up. Try a little ritual to reinforce all these bright feelings of newness—start a brand-new journal, say a little prayer, or do something you've never done before to honor the occasion.

Never Skip Two Days in a Row

When you're starting out, the first day matters. Baby steps matters. But once you've started, it's all about preserving your momentum. Momentum is nothing mysterious, though—it's simply our ability to keep moving once we've started moving. We don't need to continually maintain the same degree of intensity, though. You can slow down, only don't completely *stop*!

In the beginning, there may be a strong and perfectly natural desire to miss a day here and there. Nobody's perfect and remember, your brain is working hard to bring you back to its old equilibrium, so you may be pushing hard against the tendency to run back to your comfort zone. But once you've begun, make a promise to yourself that although you can skip a day here or there, you will never skip two days in a row.

This is a great rule to have for yourself, because it's flexible. We all mess up from time to time. Maybe you're ill. Maybe some truly unexpected emergency crops up. That's fine. If you skip a day, forgive yourself and move on—but don't allow yourself to do it again. Otherwise, you are on the path to making it a habit. One day is a normal setback. Two days starts to seriously undo your momentum.

All or nothing thinking can be deadly when we're trying to learn new habits and genuinely improve our lives. If you are ultra-strict with yourself and freak out when you're not perfect, you may actually send yourself into a downward spiral and think, "Well, I'm so far gone now I might as well give up." But you don't have to aim for perfection. You just need to be consistent—and giving up is the one thing that will destroy that consistency!

How to Use This in Your Life Immediately

Your attitude is what will make the difference.

This two-day rule is really a psychological trick. We are in essence immunizing ourselves against small setbacks and simply refusing to let them turn into big setbacks.

Step 1: When you mess up, deliberately move away from bad feelings about yourself. You haven't failed; it's not a catastrophe. In fact, it's pretty normal and one hundred percent predictable. Whatever you do, don't allow bad feelings to get in the way of you continuing your mission. Remind yourself that messing up one day is not a sign that you're a hopeless case, but simply that your approach needs adjusting. That's it. It's just data.

Step 2: Take that data and see what you can learn. What needs to change to make sure this doesn't happen again? Take the slip-up as valuable, welcome feedback. You didn't think the process of change would be perfectly smooth sailing, right?

Step 3: Set up consequences for not following through on two days. You need to really, really feel that it's impossible for you to miss two days in a row. Encourage this belief by having someone else hold you accountable, or find a way to make the consequences so real and uncomfortable that it's actually preferable just to get back onto your winning streak again.

As an example, let's say you fail to go to gym one day even though you've been the last two weeks straight. You pause and look at *why*. You don't wallow in self-pity or beat yourself up. You just say, "Hm, what happened there?" Maybe you notice that you missed your morning workout because you stayed up all night and were too exhausted. The actionable next step is clear: go to bed on time tonight and don't miss your workout tomorrow.

Monitor Your Progress

So you've broken things into baby steps, you've taken the first and most important baby step, and piece by piece, day by day, you are building your goal. Well done! Now you're well and truly on the path, you'll need to keep track of how you're going. Knowledge is power.

Tracking helps you stay focused on what's important to reaching your goal. It also helps you identify potential obstacles and strategies for how to overcome them—*before* they derail you. Consciously tracking your development can help you set more realistic goals and stay positive along the way, because you are seeing concrete evidence of your incremental improvement.

Think about keeping a journal to write down your self-discipline goals and to track your progress. Alternatively, you could have a highly visible chart somewhere to remind you of the journey you're on. This reinforces the positive changes that you're implementing in your life and gives you a record that you can look back on with pride—especially on those days you feel like giving up. It might be tempting to miss a day, but then when you look at your unbroken streak of twenty days, you might decide to push on instead of interrupting that momentum.

This is the power of tracking—if you know what your baseline is, you know, without doubt, whether your interventions are actually working and how much they're working. The simple act of measuring yourself alone is a boost of motivation. Think of it as having yourself as an accountability buddy. On the other hand, if something isn't working, tracking yourself will show you this clearly and immediately and give you a chance to identify what is actually the source and magnitude of the problem.

That takes us to the obvious question—*how* do you track?

How to Use This in Your Life Immediately

If you're thinking you need some kind of complex app or tool to get you started, hold on—the first step is actually to determine *what metrics* you can use to measure your progress. Your progress may naturally lend itself to being quantified and measured, but it may not. For example, you may be trying to lose weight, and so you could settle on measuring pounds of weight lost. However, take a moment to think about this carefully. If you only have five pounds to lose, you might choose smaller increments than one pound, or you may choose other metrics entirely, such as waist measurements or how close you are to wearing a too-tight pair of trousers!

Don't rush this step. First, zoom out and look at the bigger picture, i.e., your larger goal. Then think about realistic, appropriate time scales (again, baby steps will help here!). Reflect on why you're doing what you're doing, and then choose a frequency at which you'll check in on your progress to completing these mini-goals or baby steps. With our example, you might want to lose weight primarily for health reasons and decide that indefinitely checking in weekly makes sense since you are looking to make gradual changes that will last for the long term (i.e., you're not just crash dieting to lose weight by next Wednesday).

Once you've decided on how often you're checking in, decide on how you'll track your progress. Again, choose what is appropriate. Keep it simple. You might keep a chart on the bathroom wall where you record your weekly weigh in, joining up the dots to form a graph that shows you your progress over time. Progress tracking works best when you build in a little ritual and reward with each step. Take a moment at every interval to look at how far you've come, remind yourself where you're going, and celebrate the steps you're taking to get there.

Put Your Goals Where You Can See Them

In the above example, the tracking chart was placed visibly in the bathroom where it would be seen every day, even on those days where no actual weighing in would happen. This is no accident. You've heard the phrase, "get it in writing." Well, goals are the same—when written down, they become more real to our unconscious minds, and are more likely to be achieved. Writing goals down forces you to clarify them, put them into concrete words and *see* them out there in the world. It's the first step to making them real.

Written down goals (as well as visible tracking) are a kind of positive reinforcement. Any time we follow a desired behavior with a reinforcing stimulus, we are making that behavior more likely to occur again in the future. Ordinarily, we think of this reinforcer as a reward (e.g., having a treat after you complete an exam), but simply marking your progress has the same effect. Tracking progress against a written goal makes your achievement more tangible and allows you to enjoy it more, making positive associations between the behavior and you feeling good.

And that's the key right there: the more you can attach positive feelings to your desired actions, the more likely it is you'll keep doing those actions. For example:

- You write down an inspiring and motivational message for yourself, capturing your reason for aiming for your goal. You place this prominently in your office and look at it daily. This encourages you. Those good feelings come to be associated with working

in your office, and you find yourself *wanting* to be there and to achieve your goal.
- You have a white board in your study with your week's goals written on one side. As you complete tasks, you erase them and rewrite them on the other side. Now you have visual evidence of everything you've achieved (positive reinforcement—you're making progress!) as well as a clear indication of what's outstanding.
- You have a jar filled with pieces of paper, each with "$100" written on it. As you pay down a large debt, you manually remove the papers and tear them up, burn them, or throw them in the trash. Doing so feels so good! You reward and reinforce each one hundred dollars paid, as well as encourage yourself to keep going and empty that jar for good.

How to Use This in Your Life Immediately

Firstly, make sure you are not shaming or scaring yourself into achieving your goals. Punishments and negative emotions can control your behavior to some extent, but you're far more likely to make sustainable changes if you make the process genuinely enjoyable and meaningful. Focus on ways you can make every step of your journey as pleasurable and positive as possible. Don't underestimate the satisfaction to be found in tracking your progress. Tell yourself out loud, "I'm getting closer every day to my goal" and allow yourself to bask for a few moments in those good, encouraging feelings.

Write down your goals. Make them clear, simple, and workable. Then make sure you can *see* how you are getting closer and closer to that goal. Hang your written goals or progress charts up somewhere or put them where you can see them every single day. Use calendars, stick things to your fridge, put notes on your computer screen, or even set reminders on your phone. You can set a specific time every day to check in, perhaps noting that you've gone one more full day without (insert addictive behavior here). Pat yourself on the back.

Visualize Your Outcome
Visualization comes naturally to anyone making a goal. We've all fantasized about

what life would be like once we achieve our dream. However, visualization is not just daydreaming; it's a powerful tool that spurs and maintains our motivation. Visualization helps self-discipline because your brain can't actually differentiate between real and imagined images. So, when you imagine something vividly, your brain chemistry changes as if you're actually experiencing those images.

Visualizing positive things gives you positive feelings and associations, reinforcing your behavior and keeping you on track. This makes it easier for you to overcome feelings of fear and take actionable steps toward achieving your goals. So, dreaming and visualizing are not magical—they prepare and prompt your brain to actually achieve what you're holding in your imagination. Your motivation spikes. Your unconscious gets to work on finding creative solutions for your problems. You are programming yourself to expect a positive outcome and to recognize opportunities and possibilities in line with your dream.

It's not a question of "imagine it and it will mysteriously manifest in your life," but rather, the more clearly you can picture what you're aiming for, the more efficient you'll be at making that a reality. Athletes, for example, take pains to "rehearse" a certain move or play in their mind long before they train their physical muscles to follow through. The mental preparation lays the foundation and gives them the confidence, focus and conviction to then bring that vision to life. In the same way that an athlete actually creates new neural pathways just by thinking about a certain action, you can do the same, and start training your brain to behave as though what you want is already true in some sense.

How to Use This in Your Life Immediately

You can use visualization to imagine a detailed and vivid outcome—this inspires and motivates you and creates a degree of focus and fearlessness. *Example: imagining yourself crossing the finish line on marathon day.*

Or you could visualize the process toward your goal—this helps prepare and organize you, as well as keep you on track and help you predict and pre-empt possible obstacles. Example: mentally imagining yourself pushing through and achieving your training goals day by day. Literally picture yourself facing resistance and laziness and triumphing over it.

Visualizing is a focused, deliberate act. Close your eyes and take your time painting a mental picture of what you want to happen. Play it out like a movie in your mind. Draw on all five of your senses—imagine how the scene looks, sounds, etc.—but most importantly, sink into how you *feel* in this image. This is vital. Summon up the physical sensations in your body, the emotions you feel, as well as any words, gestures or facial expressions. This is what will really help those new neural pathways cement themselves.

You can play around with your visualization. Some people imagine the image shrinking down into a magical pill they then eat or swallow, and then visualize it going into their bodies and powering up their motivation. Others might imagine a gold frame around an imagined scene, or imbue it with a specially chosen song or mantra that transports them into just the right frame of mind. Visualization can also be done via collages or "vision boards"—collect physical pictures that capture the feeling you want to create with your goal and hang it somewhere prominent. Visualization is not just visual—you can use affirmations or specific phrases, too (for example, imagine in detail the speech you will give once you earn a coveted award, and imagine the sound of the applause).

Visualization is best done regularly. Build it into your daily routine or do it after you've achieved a goal or had a setback—it can act like a compass, keeping you on track in both cases. Remember, the image, whatever it is, must be alive and *felt* in your body to have any power.

Summary:

- When cultivating the self-discipline needed to achieve your goals, it matters how you start. Forego quantum leaps and overnight successes and instead "think small" by breaking your big goal down into manageable, sustainable baby steps. What matters most is habit and consistency.
- You have more chance of achieving your goal if you make a conscious "fresh

start," i.e., begin on New Year's Day, your birthday, or the first day of the week, Monday. Deliberately and consciously mark the occasion and make it memorable, telling yourself that the past is forgiven and forgotten, and you are turning over a new leaf.

- Make a promise to yourself that even though you may occasionally have setbacks, you will never skip your task for two days in a row. One day is understandable, but two days makes a habit. If you slip up, go into learning mode and ask why so you can ensure you don't do the same the following day.
- Choose a goal, set a timeframe, and then choose some appropriate metrics to track and monitor your progression. Keep this visible and concrete, to inspire you, give you a sense of focus and accomplishment, and help you troubleshoot and pre-empt problems.
- Finally, use the power of visualization to train your brain in the right direction. Draw on all five senses to imagine the desired outcome or the process toward that outcome—or both. What matters is

that you do it regularly and really delve into the *feelings* associated with what you're trying to create.

Chapter 2: Focus on Habits

Replace Old Habits

You've heard it all before—good habits are the foundation of a healthy, successful life. But here's the good news: you don't need to start from scratch. Think about it this way, you *already have* habits. Your brain naturally wants to do certain things on autopilot, repeatedly. You just have to make sure that the thing you're doing automatically is the best possible option for you.

Most of the time, *bad* habits are simply a way of dealing with stress and boredom. Everything from biting your nails to overspending on a shopping spree to drinking every weekend to wasting time on the internet. These are all (unhelpful) ways to regulate our emotions, manage stress, and "fill the void," whatever it may be.

But it doesn't have to be that way. You can teach yourself new and healthy ways to deal with stress and boredom, which you can then substitute in place of your bad habits. The good thing about this approach is that you already have the mental scaffolding in place, so to speak. You are merely swapping out the content of a habit you already have for something better. Can you "break" a bad habit by sheer force of will? Yes. But it takes enormous amounts of energy and focus. You can achieve the same result by replacing habits or upgrading them.

A good example is if you're trying to stop yourself shopping online when you take a break at work. This bad habit destroys your focus and attention, because you're likely to be online for twenty to thirty minutes each time. But maybe you find that every time you're tempted to shop, you're simply faced with a big gaping hole in your schedule and the unfulfilled desire to browse your favorite sites. It's an uphill battle each time. What now?

Firstly, recognize that bad habits, as harmful as they are, are serving a purpose and have some benefit in your life—otherwise, they wouldn't be there. The first step is to notice when you feel triggered or compelled to do the bad habit. Then, understand what that habit is doing for you. Releasing boredom? Acting as a welcome distraction from life stress?

You can guess what the next step is: find a new, healthier way to satisfy that need for yourself without resorting to your bad habit. In our shopping example, perhaps you recognize that you are browsing to relieve tension and "treat" yourself. After some brainstorming, you realize you can do this by taking a walk outside and indulging in a healthy snack, a book you're enjoying, or a few moments spent on a hobby. Maybe, in time, you recognize that stress levels at your job are unsustainable and that you need to make bigger changes in that area, i.e., addressing the stress or leaving the job completely.

How to Use This in Your Life Immediately

Answer the following questions to guide your bad habit replacement:

What bad habits do you have right now?

What are the where, what, who, why, and when of this habit?

What is this habit costing you and what could you regain by replacing it?

Was there a time before the bad habit? What were you like then? What did you do instead?

What is the benefit/function of this habit in your life?

What substitute behavior can give you the same feeling or outcome as this bad habit, but healthily?

What are the benefits of switching to this behavior in place of the bad behavior?

What are your bad habit triggers (think who, where, why, how...)?

Can you visualize yourself perceiving these triggers but focusing your attention on the new habit instead?

What could you do immediately afterward to reward yourself for diverting to this better habit?

Eat Well, Eat Regularly

Chances are that healthy eating is one of the habits you intend you cultivate within yourself by finding enough self-discipline and motivation. But the truth is, it may go the other way around, that is, that self-discipline is a *result* of healthy eating and not a *cause*. Your blood sugar levels are directly and closely linked to your degree of self-control and energy, which impact in a big way on how disciplined you can be in your everyday choices and actions.

Willpower is not an infinite resource and gets depleted just like anything else. The brain literally runs on glucose as a fuel, therefore if you're hungry, you're simply not going to be as focused as you possibly can be. Studies have shown that low blood sugar often weakens a person's resolve. When you're hungry, your ability to concentrate suffers as your brain is not functioning to its highest potential. Hunger makes it difficult to focus on the tasks at hand, not to mention making you grumpy and pessimistic.

Now, a caveat here: eating a healthy diet is not about strict limitations, staying unrealistically thin, or depriving yourself of the foods you love. Rather, it's about feeling great, having more energy, improving your health, and boosting your mood. To set yourself up for success, try to keep things simple. Food really is fuel, and when you're making changes to your life and cultivating discipline, you need that energy, and you need to eat strategically.

Eating a healthier diet doesn't have to be complicated. But you do need a few key rules to live by, to guide you. Instead of being overly concerned with counting calories, for example, think of your diet in terms of color, variety, and freshness. Focus on avoiding packaged and processed foods and opting for more fresh ingredients whenever possible. Avoid snacks, eat when you're hungry and stop when you're full, and stay away from foods that actively harm you, like alcohol or loads of refined sugar and salt.

Having food rules is not about being on a diet or adopting restrictive eating. It's more about applying your own values and principles to this super important area of life and taking responsibility for what you put in your mouth. In a way, it doesn't matter all that much what your food rules are, only that they matter to you, that they are sustainable, and that they consistently allow you to achieve the health and balance you want. Michael Pollan, food journalist and author of *The Omnivore's Dilemma*, has his own three-part food rule: "Eat real food (i.e., not processed rubbish), mostly plants, not too much." Simple, huh?

How to Use This in Your Life Immediately

What food rules will work for your life? There is a matter of trial and error, but as far as self-discipline is concerned, the best diet is one that is varied, balanced, and *steady*. Keep your blood sugar levels as constant as possible and eat a wide range of foods at regular intervals. Avoid bingeing or long fast periods. Take a look at some of these other popular food rules that have served people for centuries and see which can be slotted effectively into your life:

- Eat some protein with every meal

- Have at least five servings of fruit and veggies a day, all different colors

- Home cook most of your meals from scratch

- Drink plenty of water

- Avoid anything with the fiber removed, i.e., opt for brown rice and wholewheat pasta instead of white

- Replace bread, pastry, pasta, and cakes with starchy vegetables

- No food is off limits—it's all about moderation and portion control

- Cut down on meat and eat more fish and veggie sources of protein

- Eat less salt and sugar, and don't add any to your meals

- Eat until you're seventy percent full, eat slowly, and chew well

- A little treat now and then won't kill you!

Exercise Body . . . and Mind

We couldn't mention healthy eating without also mentioning the value of regular physical movement and exercise. The two go hand in hand when it comes to creating a solid foundation onto which you can start building success and achieving your dreams.

This point is all about the following maxim: **how you do anything is how you do everything.** How does physical exercise benefit your overall discipline? If you exercise regularly, your willpower muscle will be stronger, too. When you exercise your physical body, you are also training your strength of will and dedication. You are teaching yourself that you can and will follow through on your commitments, and training your ability to stick it out and get it done.

Exercise is a precious cornerstone to a life filled with good and positive habits and free from bad habits. Not only is it brilliant for your physical health, but it will keep your mental health in tip-top form as well, helping you feel confident, capable, and energized as you move through your day. Instill the keystone habit of exercise into your morning routine, and you turbo charge each day with enthusiasm and focus right from the beginning. Plus, you get to tick something significant off your list and feel the sense of accomplishment that brings.

Exercise reliably reduces your levels of stress and pain by releasing endorphins and neurotransmitters such as dopamine and serotonin. Exercise improves total health by increasing blood flow and the oxygenation of the body's cells, toning the immune system, and helping it fight off diseases. Your mood will improve, you'll sleep better, and maybe, just maybe, you'll look better naked!

Again, regular physical exercise is the result of self-discipline, but it is also its cause. When you practice discipline in one area of your life, it's inevitable that your dedication will spill over into other areas, too.

How to Use This in Your Life Immediately

As with so many other things in life, don't overthink it. Start small and stay consistent. If you're starting from zero, the most important thing is to clarify exactly what you want to achieve—not all of us can be fitness models (or want to be). Once you're clear on what you want and why you want it, then set a single, realistic, quantifiable goal for yourself; for example, to get through a one-hour HIIT workout class. Then, assign yourself regular tasks throughout the week—it's best if your workout happens at the same, non-negotiable time of day, every day. Naturally, you want to choose a time when you're most wired up and ready to move.

In the beginning, just focus on what's directly in front of you: that day's workout, that set, that rep. Focus on the immediate short-term gains, not the big transformations you're hoping to ultimately achieve. Simply notice that you feel good after getting your blood flowing. Reward yourself, track your progress, and let it sink in that you're on the path. Always have a *plan*. At all times, you need to know exactly what exercise is lined up for you in the future—don't leave it up to willpower alone, but schedule it in.

Eat well, sleep enough, and get the people in your life on board so they can support you. Avoid temptations and be kind to yourself—slipping up is part of the process, but don't dwell on it. Just get back on the wagon and carry on as soon as you can.

Finally, a note about the kind of exercise you should try. That's simple: pick something that you can genuinely imagine yourself doing day in and day out. You don't *have to* do weight training or skipping or jogging or whatever. Choose something you love and which challenges you. That could be yoga, dance, swimming, mountain climbing, or whatever else floats your boat. Just make sure that a) you're moving your body, and b) you're doing it every single day.

Fine Tune Your Mornings

You're probably beginning to notice a theme here! Self-discipline, motivation, organization, and commitment to achieving your goals sound like vague, abstract things "out there" in the world, but the truth is, successful living starts *in here*, with your body and with your everyday routines. In other words, no goal is so ethereal and lofty that it can override a lack of sleep, a diet of junk food or a bad drinking habit. Willpower is not going to get you very far if you are not giving yourself a solid physiological foundation on which to build.

With that in mind, let's turn now to arguably one of the best routines to nail down in your mission to become the most productive, most self-disciplined version of yourself: your wake-up time. Consider it an extension of the idea that *how you do anything is how you do everything*. It's not rocket science—how you start the day is usually an indication of how the rest of your day is going to pan out. It works both ways: a person who is disciplined and motivated will have no trouble getting up and on with the day ahead, and a person who can manage to wake up consistently at the right time will find that they naturally feel more motivated and disciplined with everything that follows.

The key, surprise surprise, is consistency and commitment. As your first act of the day, prove to yourself that you have the self-control, agency and sense of purpose to get up and get moving. Rather than letting your day start without you or falling into your routine almost by accident, seize it consciously and deliberately, putting your own intention into the way that events unfold from the second you open your eyes.

How to Use This in Your Life Immediately

Let's look at the facts first—human beings naturally move through a twenty-four-hour wake/sleep cycle, with rising and falling energy and concentration levels. While each of us has a different "chronotype" i.e., personal biological rhythm, the truth is that *everyone* needs at least seven hours of sleep (eight is better) and *everyone* is happier and healthier when they wake up and go to sleep at a consistent time every day—including on the weekends!

If you're like most people, you're in the bad habit of staying up too late at night and then struggling to get up early enough in the morning. If so, your aim is two-fold—gradually inch your bedtime and your wake time earlier, and once they're where you want them, maintain them using positive reinforcement. Making big changes to your current schedule won't last; instead, shift your routine by fifteen minutes at a time, for as few days at a time, before shifting it again.

An early bedtime goes hand in hand with an early morning. So, while you're training yourself to wake up on time, spend equal amounts of energy on tidying up your nighttime routine:

Have a "wind down" routine where you take a hot bath, do yoga, journaling, reading, meditating, or listening to relaxing music for the hour before you sleep. Consciously release the stress and thoughts of the day and get ready to sleep, ensuring that your room is as dark, quiet, and comfortable as possible. Even if you don't fall asleep, that's fine. Just rest. Whatever you do, don't stare at pixelated, glowing screens in the hour before bed.

In the morning, put your alarm clock somewhere where you'll need to get up to turn it off. The moment your alarm goes off, communicate to your body that it's time for wakefulness:

- Open the window to let in natural light and fresh air
- Make your bed so you're not tempted to get back into it
- Enjoy some movement—a nice walk outside, stretching, or anything you like to wake your body up

Stick to a Schedule

Here's something to get your head around: setting up a fixed daily routine and following a schedule is not hard work. It's actually the *easy way*. When you stick to tried-and-true routines and get into the habit of following an organized schedule, there's simply less to think about, and you require *less* willpower, not more. Habit and automation are the secret superpower of all successful people. Routines make the best use of our time, cut down on indecision and overwhelm, boost our confidence and feeling of achievement, get a good momentum going, and free up our minds to do more creative, novel work.

Motivation and inspiration are great, but it's consistency and discipline that will keep you on the path even when motivation is flagging. What's the best schedule? One that is written down. The act of writing out and contemplating your routine solidifies it and makes it more likely that you'll follow through.

How to Use This in Your Life Immediately

Sit down with a pen and paper. Outline the seven days of the week. First add in your wake and sleep times and block out enough time for sleep. Then, schedule in your morning and evening routine—say roughly and hour for each. You can include things like stretching, having a good breakfast, reading, visualization, walking, tidying your home, grooming, and so on.

Go back to the goals you have identified for yourself, break them down into smaller chunks, and schedule them in. Remember to give yourself ample time for breaks, time to digest and consolidate, time to reflect on what you've done, and time to plan ahead. Don't leave this up to chance—schedule it in and protect that time!

Give yourself time for meals and exercise and play around with your allotted time so that you are giving every area of your life the attention it deserves. You might like to have a general schedule, but fine tune it every Sunday evening where you plan in more detail according to what's going on in your life. But in this case, your morning and evening routines should still stay as consistent as humanly possible.

Sounds good right? Let's actually make it happen, though:

- Make sure that everything is written down and visible to you every day.
- Build your schedule around your priorities and non-negotiables. Only you can identify these for yourself.
- When you have many smaller tasks like chores and admin, cluster them together.
- Pay attention to your own peak energy and concentration times and schedule the most difficult or demanding task for then.
- Keep in mind all the things you *won't* do, and don't allow yourself to get distracted or sidetracked. Don't multitask.
- Your routine is not set in stone—stay flexible so that when you review

(which you should be doing at least weekly), you can make intelligent adjustments that reflect real life and have the best chance of actually working for you. The "perfect" schedule is worthless if it's not realistically doable.

I want to mention two important things here that you might not pay much attention to when you're drawing up your schedule. The first is patience, and the second is forgiveness. The fact is, while a routine makes life easier once it's established, habits take time to embed themselves in your life, and you will need patience until then. Secondly, you will mess up. Be realistic. Life is messy and seldom plays out in discrete, predictable chunks. If you can't follow your schedule now and then, don't beat yourself up. Mitigate the unexpected, flow around the interruption, and keep going. If you're routinely finding that your schedule just doesn't work, that's not a sign to give up, but a sign that you need to make some careful adjustments.

Make Room for Breaks, Treats, and Rewards

When most people start out with making a schedule, they think solely of work. They block in their paid employment and then, consciously or unconsciously, allow themselves the scraps of time around those hours to somehow live the rest of their lives. Kind of depressing when you think about it, right?

Living a more self-disciplined life doesn't mean you need to live like your own drill sergeant, completely rigid and inflexible, unforgiving, punishing, and joyless. In fact, trying to achieve this is likely to make you less resilient and far less productive in the long run. Zero wiggle room often results in failures, disappointments, and giving in to your old ways. In other words, being too extreme is not particularly sustainable.

Breaks are important. Your rest and recuperation and joy in life is important. For its own sake, but also because it will make you a more focused, whole and motivated person overall. Breaks, treats, and rewards cement and acknowledge your progress and keep your motivation up. Here's how to make use of them:

How to Use This in Your Life Immediately

Make rewards appropriate. This is obvious—your reward should not undermine or cancel out your achievement. It should also be significant enough to actually mean something to you and should be something you genuinely like and want. Make sure you know exactly when you will be rewarded, and when you reach that milestone, pause and truly relish the joy of your success. Brag a little, honor the occasion, and share your pride. Let the good feelings sink in—they will actively rewire your brain for success and release dopamine, which is a powerful reward neurotransmitter that will make the preceding behavior more likely to be repeated.

If you've lost some weight, don't reward yourself with half a cake and a skipped workout—you are only reversing your progress and telling yourself that you actually prefer to eat poorly and neglect your physical health. Instead, tell yourself how good it feels to live healthily and treat yourself to a massage, a new gadget you've had your eye on, or an afternoon off catching up with a loved one.

Rewards and treats don't have to be material and don't have to cost a lot of money. A good idea is to make a list of things that give you joy and reinvigorate your purpose and passion. Consult this list when your energy is flagging and you need a pick-me-up. Getting outdoors, socializing with others, enjoying good food and music, moving your body, having a hot bath, snuggling up a with a book or a podcast, or simply trying something new are all great ways to healthily treat and reward your progress.

Get the most from your breaks. Schedule them in like they're important appointments (they are!) and don't be tempted to skip over them. A good rule of thumb when working is to have a full break every forty minutes to an hour for around ten minutes. Have a longer break (twenty minutes) for every four hours you work. Make sure you're never sitting down like a lump for extended periods. Pepper your day with movement and keep things varied.

Get up, stretch your legs, have a hot cup of tea, go outside for a while, chat to a friend, engage in a hobby, have a micro nap or have a healthy snack to replenish your blood sugar. Inject some mindfulness into every one of your breaks and check in with yourself—are your eyes getting strained and need a break? Are you slouching? Hungry? Maybe you need to switch task and come back to a problem later, after letting your unconscious mind chew on it for a while.

Summary:

- To become more disciplined, focus on your bad habits and work not to eliminate them but replace them with better ones. Observe your current habits, understand the purpose they serve, their triggers and their results, and take action to rework them in your favor. With good habits in place, you need *less* self-discipline, not more.
- It sounds basic, but you cannot cultivate self-discipline without the foundation of a healthy lifestyle. You can fuel your willpower by considering how to fuel your body first. There are many different diet philosophies, and they all work, but one thing consistently shown

to improve self-control is to maintain stable blood sugar levels.
- Regular exercise will boost your self-esteem, fill your body with endorphins, keep you fit and strong, and help you exercise your resolve as you exercise your muscles. Remember: how you do anything is how you do everything. Exercise not only your body but your mind.
- If you don't have one already, establish a rock-solid morning routine that gets you started on the right foot. Each person has their own unique biorhythms, but most of us benefit from having regular sleep and wake times and healthy sleep habits.
- Give yourself less work to do by having a weekly schedule, which is built around your priorities. Cluster less important tasks together and build in some wiggle room and time to appraise and adjust.
- Make sure you are scheduling in ample time to rest and recuperate, as well as time to acknowledge your progress and reward yourself. This is crucial for your ongoing success!

Chapter 3: Get Right in Your Body, Mind and Soul

Remove Temptations

In the last chapter, we looked at ways to lay the all-important foundations of a self-disciplined life, including healthy habits with sleep, exercise and diet. In this chapter, we'll turn our attention to the impact that our attitude, our moods, and our thought processes have on our ability to self-regulate and take control of our lives. So many of us know what we should be doing and *want* to do it, yet we falter time and again when tempted or distracted by things in our environment.

You need self-discipline. But this doesn't mean bravely wrestling it out and pitching your willpower up against very tempting prospects. To be honest, this rarely works, and even if it does, your willpower will eventually deplete, whereas there's no end to the number of temptations and distractions out there, ready to derail your progress. No, if we hope to reduce the effect of these temptations on our lives, we need to be smart about it. We need to manage, pre-empt, or flat-out avoid those moments where we are vulnerable to throwing our resolve out the window.

Self-control is often easiest when abiding by the old saying, "out of sight, out of mind." Removing all temptations and distractions from your environment is essential. Set up systems that remove the necessity of willpower in the first place, in other words, make doing the bad things tough, and make doing the good things easy—or even automatic.

How to Use This in Your Life Immediately

Step 1: Be honest. When you're fired up with a new goal you might not be inclined to think of potential setbacks, but you control them best when you are fully aware of what they are, where they come from, when and how. The idea is to make sure that you have a solid strategy *before* you are staring at the temptation in the moment. When you set a goal, identify your potential temptations and triggers to quit. Be honest with yourself about how enticing they'll be!

Step 2: Avoid. You don't have to do anything about temptation if you are never actually faced with it, right? So just avoid. Alternatively, fight distractions with more distraction—if you have a mad craving for sugar one day, just make sure you're entertaining yourself for the next ten minutes and putting yourself far out of the reach of any tempting treats. Then, even if you succumb to the craving and decide to go for it—you physically cannot. Your resolve will return, and the craving will pass. Make sure you're distracting yourself until then. If you can't avoid the temptation, then reduce and mitigate it. If you can't avoid going to that restaurant, at least plan ahead and commit to ordering the best thing off the menu before you even arrive, and turn down the dessert menu.

Step 3: Visualize. Plan ahead how you will respond to inevitable temptations by rehearsing what you'll do. Literally close your eyes and play out the scene in your mind. Picture yourself in vivid detail turning away from the temptation. Then, importantly, imagine yourself feeling really good afterward, confident and encouraged that you were able to push through. Visualizing this way helps cancel out a big reason we so often fail—we forget about the future and the long-term consequences of our choices. Remind yourself of why you're doing what you're doing, and really feel that the temporary pleasure doesn't compare to the sense of satisfaction you'll feel from achieving your goal.

The great thing about temptation is that it's fleeting. Bad habit, physical craving, and plain old boredom can feel super powerful in the moment, but they really aren't. Resisting them means losing out on that moment of pleasure. But if you can do it, you gain so much more. You gain momentum (next time, resisting will be easier), confidence and pride in yourself, encouragement, and the knowledge that you have just taken one more crucial step toward the thing you *really* want: your goal.

Don't Wait for it to "Feel Right"

Well, resisting temptation is a valuable skillset. But sometimes, what threatens to derail the best laid plan is nothing—by that I mean simply procrastinating or avoiding what you need to do. Getting into a disciplined, proactive state of mind means looking frankly at the beliefs and assumptions that are keeping us stuck and encouraging us to be less than we could be.

If procrastination and avoidance are something you battle with, then what may be to blame is the unconscious belief that you can only take action when you're feeling inspired and motivated to do so. And unless you're ultra-energized and enthusiastic, then you have to wait for a better time to start. The truth is, motivation is not necessary. To achieve your goals, you need only keep on taking daily action toward them. That's it. Some days you'll feel jazzed up and ready to go, some days you won't. But discipline means showing up and doing the work regardless of the fleeting ebbs and flows of enthusiasm.

Another way to think of it is that action causes enthusiasm, rather than the other way around. If you take action, you inspire and motivate yourself, not to mention feel encouraged and proud of yourself. Keep procrastinating, though, and your self-esteem will only plummet further, and it'll start to feel harder and harder to get going again.

Nothing bad will happen to you if you do things you're uncomfortable with, or things that don't exactly light your world on fire. Seriously, it won't hurt you. Charles Duhigg, author of *The Power of Habit*, explains that habit behaviors are traced to a part of the brain called the basal ganglia, which is associated with emotions, patterns, and memories. Decisions, on the other hand, are made in the prefrontal cortex, a completely different area.

When a behavior becomes habit, we stop using our decision-making skills and instead function on autopilot. Therefore, breaking a bad habit and building a new habit not only requires us to make active decisions, it will feel wrong. Your brain will resist the change in favor of what it has been programmed to do. The solution? Embrace the wrong. Acknowledge that it will take a while for your new regime to feel right or good or natural. Keep chugging along. It will happen. Don't assume that fear or listlessness or inertia mean that you're on the wrong path—most likely, the opposite is true!

It can be a relief to know that ending procrastination has nothing to do with willpower or laziness. It can be managed with a few simple behavioral tricks.

How to Use This in Your Life Immediately

One surefire tip? Just start. Tell yourself all that matters is doing five minutes, or even one minute. You don't have to *like* it, just get started. Don't plan or overthink, just begin. Then notice once you've started that it's not so bad! Stop telling yourself to wait for the right moment, and stop saying "I don't have the time." You do. And the right time is now.

If your energy is genuinely low and you're procrastinating because you doubt your ability to do the task well, then work on managing your energy levels—not the task itself. Break it down and schedule small chunks for your peak energy times in the day. Do an easier task first to get the ball rolling, if you must. It may sound counterproductive, but have a break. Make it a real break, not just a stressful exercise in avoidance where you're just thinking about the upcoming task.

If procrastination is more serious or chronic, however, your job is to dig deep and find out *why* you're procrastinating. Fear of failure? Fear of success? Working on a goal you don't actually care about? Other people's expectations? Perfectionism? Once you've identified the thoughts and beliefs behind your procrastination, you can take a more targeted approach to fixing it.

Focus on the Positive

Remember dopamine, your brain's reward chemical? You are far more likely to make positive changes in your life, to be productive and effective and successful, if you do so with a positive, healthy frame of mind. Self-improvement is not about punishment, shame or deprivation. It's not about hating or judging yourself into being better. There are two reasons to bring more compassion and positivity to the change process:

1. You'll be more resilient to setbacks, obstacles and failure,
2. You'll enjoy it more!

When you fail or mess up (notice that it's when and not if), you will need to respond with self-compassion. Think of it this way: beating yourself up achieves precisely nothing and will not get you back on the wagon. What will get you back on the path is to gently forgive yourself, become curious about what happened and why, and then take intelligent action to do better next time. But the important first step is the compassion.

Instituting a new way of thinking won't always go according to plan. You will have ups and downs, fabulous successes, and flat-out failures. The key is to keep moving forward whatever the situation is. It will be a journey, and you won't always perform as you'd ideally like. That's perfectly normal. It's easy to get wrapped up in guilt, anger, or frustration, but these emotions will not improve self-discipline. In fact, they could make you feel so bad that you're tempted to give up entirely. Instead, use the hiccups in your plan as learning experiences for the future. Forgive yourself, focus on the positive, and get back in the saddle ASAP. The longer you're off your game, the harder it is to keep going in a positive direction.

A positive mindset is a resilient, flexible, living one. It's what allows you to learn and evolve. It's what makes it possible to face a challenge or setback square on and say, "Okay. That's fine. What can I do now? What have I learned?"

How to Use This in Your Life Immediately

There are dozens of practical ways that you can start including more positivity and self-compassion in your life, today.

- Practice gratitude. Every day note a few things you're thankful for, and dwell for a moment on everything that's going right for you.
- Stay in the present. Often, negative thinking is all about the past or the future. Try to notice when you're ruminating on what's happened or worrying about what will happen, and gently bring your mind to the present instead. The present, after all, is where all the possibilities and opportunities lie!
- Surround yourself with positive people, and avoid chronic complainers, people who sap your

energy or eternally apathetic or pessimistic people.
- Practice saying affirmations or inspirational to yourself. For example, "Success is not final; failure is not fatal. It is the courage to continue that counts."
- Look for the lesson. Mistakes are redeemed when we're brave enough to learn from them and be better next time. Then, you may even welcome failure, since it becomes a teacher.
- Drop judgment for yourself. You're not perfect, but you don't have to be. Focus not on your achievements but on your attitude and state of mind. Commit to being compassionate with yourself regardless of outcome.
- Give yourself time every day to relax, reflect and meditate. Tune into your inner voice—and not the voice of others telling you what you should and shouldn't do. Tell yourself that you always have value as a human being no matter your external achievements. What matters is not the setback but your response to it.

Mind Your Mood

We already know that your mood and your mindset can be powerful influencers over your actions. However, we do not need to be slaves to our shifting moods, or, as we already discovered, wait until we "feel like it." Self-discipline is the act of doing what your conscious intention wants to do, rather than passively allowing the whims of your mood to dictate your actions. It's a question of "mind over mood."

You can judge any situation in two main ways:

- A logical criterion. The mind.
- An emotional criterion. The mood.

Self-discipline is the conscious decision to make a mindful, logical evaluation of the facts, and then to act accordingly, even if you don't feel like it. Lack of self-discipline is the unconscious decision to make an emotional evaluation of the facts, ignore logic, and then to respond in an emotional manner according to how you feel in the moment.

Emotions are incredibly valuable. They are a guidance system in their own right and add color and depth and meaning to life. But "mood" is much simpler than this, and less reliable. When you're sitting in front of the TV and feel too lazy to get up, so you watch another episode rather than get up to clean the kitchen, that's a mood. When you are faced with something good for you but you're nervous, that's a mood. When you're cranky and fed up after a long day, that's a mood. But you don't have to allow any mood to determine what you do with your life. There's nothing wrong with having moods, and psychologically healthy people experience a range of emotions. The trick is not to let your moods be the *primary* determinant of your behavior.

It's like this: we all feel scared, or lazy or angry or tired sometimes. It's part of life. But we also possess the ability to be conscious of ourselves on another level. We can choose to zoom out and become aware of what we're feeling and act deliberately toward goals we have rationally identified as good for us. This means that we can choose to override those moods. Like temptation, moods pass. But with self-discipline, commitment, and a long-term outlook, we remain steadfast and stable through it all. We achieve our goals, despite life's ups and downs, despite the rise and fall of energy and motivation, despite setbacks or even tragedies. Because we are able to go into our logical minds and prioritize the actions we've committed to. This is very powerful.

How to Use This in Your Life Immediately

Firstly, getting a handle on moods does *not* mean squashing down emotions. But it does mean moving from a "hot" state to a "cool" one, where you are able to acknowledge what you're feeling, understand that you are in fact simply experiencing a fleeting emotional sensation, and then make room for your calmer, more rational mind to step in and remind you of your larger, long-term goals.

It's a question of lowering reactivity—i.e., learning to experience emotions and letting them pass without needing to react to them, or letting them dominate your actions. You don't need to let your emotions drag you around—*you can choose how you act regardless of how you feel.*

You don't need to become a soul-less robot; rather, become like a Zen monk who sees emerging shifts and changes in your inner emotional landscape, but without ever forgetting themselves or losing consciousness. Here are some ways to do just that:

1. Monitor yourself. When you're in a mood, it can seem like that's how you've always felt, but this is an illusion. Keep a journal where you track your changing moods so you can concretely see that moods will always shift. Your commitments and conviction, however, are more solid.
2. Notice what is making your moods worse or more volatile. As you track, notice if poor eating habits, stress or general ill health are exacerbating mood swings. Then use your rational mind to pre-empt, plan and strategize ways around that.
3. Finally, meditate. You don't need to sit cross legged like that Zen monk, but spend time in gentle contemplation, relaxation, and

turning within. The only way to master your emotions is to understand them and work with them.

Lower Other Life Stressors

If you monitor your moods for any length of time, you'll probably notice that there is an inexorable link between your overall state of health and wellbeing, and your ability to be focused, calm, and self-disciplined. This seems blindingly obvious when said out loud, but so many of us push and push and try our hardest to rekindle self-discipline all whilst undermining ourselves with our lifestyle choices and health habits—and yes, stress is perhaps the most important lifestyle factor affecting not only your health but your ability to commit to good habits.

It's simple: being stressed saps cognitive and psychological resources that you could better put to use achieving the goals you care about. If you have less to think and worry about, you have more headspace to devote to self-discipline.

Many potential stressors we face involve events or situations that require us to make changes in our ongoing lives and require time as we adjust to those changes. These changes can be positive, such as a new marriage, a planned pregnancy, a promotion, or a new house. Or they can be negative, such as the death of a loved one or a divorce. The thing is, if you are busy mitigating and managing these big changes, you will be less able to instigate any new ones, i.e., it will be far harder for you to find the energy and wherewithal for personal development of any kind.

Stress is not necessarily a bad thing—in the right amounts, it keeps us on our toes, challenges us, and keeps us honest. While no one can avoid all stress (and nobody needs to), you can work to consciously manage your stress levels in healthy, proactive ways.

How to Use This in Your Life Immediately

You've probably heard about the importance of stress management a thousand times in your life already. Maybe you know that you ought to take breaks or meditate or do a deep breathing exercise now and then. But the truth is, stress management is less a single activity or event and more a *way* of conducting every activity and event in your life. Pausing your breakneck, high-stress workday to meditate for ten minutes before hurtling right back into the fray will obviously do little to genuinely lower your stress.

One thing to bear in mind: stress management is not something you do as a "treat" or reward, it's not being lazy, and it's not optional. If stress is not managed, it will undermine your efforts to reach your goals and dampen your self-discipline, not to mention weaken your body's immunity and make life a little more miserable all around. Stress management is also not something you do only once you're *already* stressed—it's not a Band-Aid to stick on after you've already depleted your inner resources. Instead, it's something you do routinely, as part of the foundation of health and wellness that will support your grander efforts.

- You've been doing stress management all along if you have a regular exercise routine and a healthy diet that nourishes you.
- Your physical body is stressed by things like caffeine, tobacco and alcohol, and this can reflect in mental

and emotional stress, and impact your ability to recover and be resilient.
- Protect another precious resource: your time. If demands from work or family stress you, your task may be to develop healthy boundaries and to assert your own needs. Block out time everyday where you rest and recuperate, and don't allow anyone or anything to impinge on that.
- Chronic stress may be a bigger warning flag that your entire life needs a change. Ask if your ongoing stress is a sign of you not living your real values, over-compromising, or staying in a relationship or job that's not ultimately working for you.

The Emotional Eating Cycle (And How to Apply it to Other Situations)

It's hard work, getting your body, heart and soul aligned and all pulling in the same direction: toward the things that you're trying to create for yourself. Stress, temptation, bad attitudes, addictions, and negative self-talk can throw you off course just as surely as physical illness or practical constraints—if not more so.

Most people who crave more self-discipline have some sort of issue with food, either overeating or failing to stick to the healthy diet they know is best for them, and eating garbage instead. Even if "emotional eating" is not a problem for you, chances are you have a similar dynamic elsewhere in your life. As with all things, we can change these old patterns and habits by bringing our awareness to them, then taking conscious, committed action to changing them.

Food cravings are intense, sometimes irresistible urges to eat foods that are unhealthy, i.e., those high in sugar, fat or refined carbohydrates. The thing is, emotional eating is *not* a question of willpower. The foods you crave release feel-good chemicals like serotonin, dopamine, and other relaxing endorphins in your brain. These chemicals bring relief, comfort, happiness, and calmness, but they also undermine our health and, in the longer term, create havoc in the body. Because these chemicals are part of the brain's neurochemical reward system, the pleasure we feel when eating them make us more likely to seek them out again. This is the cycle—we eat those foods again, every time reinforcing the behavior.

How to Use This in Your Life Immediately

Today, these foods have been engineered in a lab to be as addictive as possible—your body literally cannot help but be drawn to them. However, you *can* beat cravings by tweaking your mindset and altering how both your body and your mind see these foods. Researchers from Brown University used MRI scans to examine the brain activity of obese or overweight study participants as they looked at pictures of drool-worthy foods like pizza, French fries, and ice cream. The researchers then tested a few different strategies, encouraging participants to focus on them for about a minute at a time. In a series of tests, they told them to:

- Get distracted by thinking about something other than food.
- Accept and allow their thoughts as something they didn't need to act on.

- Focus on the negative long-term consequences of eating those goodies.

The results? All the above allowed the participants to reduce their cravings—something that could be seen visibly in the brain itself. To apply these findings to your own life, think of it this way: submitting to cravings is a habit, and you need to replace it with a better habit. Literally train yourself so that every time you see a bad snack food, you tell yourself, "That's nice, but so what? Nobody ever died of a craving. It'll pass," and then immediately divert your attention elsewhere. Perhaps you can look at that tasty morsel and see it for what it is: a sense of disappointment in yourself, a sugar headache, and the feeling of your trousers being too tight to close the next morning. Is *that* what you want to choose?

One final secret to beating cravings for good is to understand that emotional eating is often an attempt at self-soothing, and an externalized way to emotionally regulate. If you find yourself reaching for junk food, pause and take note. What emotional need are you trying to satisfy? Then think of a healthier, more sustainable choice. If you're stressed or sad, is a sugary treat *really* going to make you feel better? What are you *really* hungry for?

Sip Some Lemonade!

Nope, this tip is not a metaphor—you can boost your self-discipline by literally drinking a little bit of lemonade. Research detailed in the APA's *Monitor on Psychology* report finds a direct link between brain glucose levels and self-control. Basically, when your glucose levels are high, you perform better on tests of self-control. This makes sense—glucose is your brain's fuel. And your self-control originates in your prefrontal cortex, which is responsible for decision making, strategizing, and planning. This means you can think of glucose as a chemical analogue for willpower.

The idea is to maintain your brain glucose levels in the ideal range so that you are always perfectly primed to make the best decisions, and act with self-restraint and conscious choice. When your brain's glucose is depleted (or too high, for that matter!) your willpower is compromised. The solution? Keep your glucose levels just right by sipping lemonade, especially during stressful or difficult times.

This may fly in the face of many assumptions around self-control. If you have a vision of self-discipline that looks like fasting and deprivation, rest assured that the science suggests otherwise. That simple glass of lemonade (or other sweet drink) can give you physical strength, which converts to better mental and psychological coping. Constant self-control depletes glucose levels, but they can be restored by that delicious glass of lemonade.

How to Use This in Your Life Immediately

Of course, this isn't an excuse to go guzzling soda or indulging in mountains of sweet treats in the name of caring for your brain. This will only have the opposite effect: dramatic peaks and dips in your blood sugar will result in headaches, energy crashes, and cranky moods. So, sadly, eating a dozen donuts won't give you God-like levels of willpower. The trick is not to maintain high blood sugar, but to keep it *steadily in the optimal zone.*

So, avoid fasting and make sure that you're eating foods with a low glycemic index and plenty of fiber, so your blood sugar levels are stable. Go for a greater number of smaller meals throughout the day instead of a few enormous ones, and avoid refined carbohydrates that will flood your body with sugar and lead to insulin spikes and drops. Make sure your meals are balanced and contain fats, good carbohydrates, and protein.

You don't need to have a full meal to replenish your glucose levels, however. Sipping lemonade provides an immediate source of glucose for your brain—take a sip or two and carry on. If you like, try sweetened tea or a small snack of fruit. Can candy and chocolate have the same effect? Yes, but these treats will also bring loads of additional calories and have a more chaotic or extreme effect on your blood sugar, not to mention you'll be falling into the same emotional eating trap outlined above.

If you find yourself dipping mood- and energy-wise during the day, just pause and become aware. Forego reaching for candy or junk food and instead breathe deeply, take a break, and get your mind right. Have a little sip of lemonade and give your brain a helping hand.

Summary:

- Getting right in body, mind, and soul means adopting the attitudes and mindsets that make a self-disciplined life possible. Firstly, make a plan to reduce, remove, and avoid temptations. If you are proactive and pre-empt them, they have less impact on your life.
- One of the biggest and most damaging myths is that we can only take action when the time is right or when we feel like it. The truth is that we can act even if we don't have the motivation! Just start, and you'll find that it's the other way around: taking action inspires you.
- Don't beat yourself up—nobody every improved from a position of judgment and self-hate. Have compassion for yourself, be kind, forgive slip-ups, and keep focusing on the positives. You do not need to make yourself feel bad in order to improve.
- We all have moods that change and shift, but we also possess the ability to choose how we respond. We can allow ourselves to feel what we feel without

letting moods disrupt our goals or commitment. Notice your moods as moods and choose not to react to them. Act instead from your rational, conscious mind.
- Willpower is a limited resource that can get depleted on the many tiny stressors and tensions of daily life. Lower your overall life stress and you free up more mental bandwidth to spend on what's really important. Stress management should be a regular habit and not reserved for when you're already struggling.
- Finally, think of glucose as the physical analogue of willpower. Sip something sweet to replenish glucose (which your brain runs on) and you improve your self-control—just make sure you're not overindulging in unhealthy sweet things.

Chapter 4: The Attitude of Success

Stop Calling Laziness Productivity

We've looked at both the physical and psychological foundations of rock-solid self-discipline, as well as the daily habits and routines that will ensure you maintain consistency and commitment until you reach your goals. Only once these fundamentals are in place can we start to talk about productivity and success. In this chapter, we'll look at self-discipline one level up—i.e., on the cognitive level. Again, though, the tips and tricks we're considering here will be ineffective if you haven't consolidated the previous levels.

You may already be someone who has a healthy lifestyle and good habits but nevertheless struggles with self-discipline and productivity. This chapter is for you. The first thing: make sure you don't get stuck in the illusion that you're being disciplined and productive when you're actually just wasting your time. While no one likes admitting it, sheer laziness is the number-one contributor to lost productivity. In fact, several so-called time-saving methods—take meetings and emails, for example, are just ways to get out of doing actual work. Place your focus on doing the things that *actually matter* most as efficiently and effectively as possible.

How do you know whether something is actually helping you reach your goals or not? Well, you look at the data. You monitor yourself, you stay conscious and accountable, and you remain willing to change and adjust according to what you find. In an attempt to be more productive, many people immediately default to what they think they *should* be doing. They start a bullet journal or force themselves to wake up at 4 a.m. because they heard some tech billionaire does it. Maybe they set up an elaborate system of "organization" that, in all honesty, is a distraction and diversion away from simply getting on with work. Similarly, if you're getting carried away with "research" and prep or you can't seem to get started until you install all the right apps and buy all the right tools, then be honest with yourself: these are not ways forward but just more the same. More laziness.

How to Use This in Your Life Immediately

The answer, as always, is to gain more conscious awareness over what is actually unfolding in each moment. As we saw in the section on building routines, you need to consistently take the time to appraise and assess your progress, to ask what's working and what isn't and why, and to make intelligent next steps to adjust your process.

Focus on one thing at a time, and pay attention to how you feel, and what results you're getting. Stay organized. Keep asking yourself this all-important question: *is what I'm doing now actively moving me forward toward my goal? Or am I stalling or going backward?*

Resistance and procrastination can take many forms, and sometimes a failure to truly act can look like fake busyness on projects that are ultimately meaningless. The process of digging to the root of your procrastination or laziness (we should really start referring to laziness as what it really is: a coping mechanism) will take time, as well as trial and error. But we need to be deadly honest about all those things that feel like positive steps but are actually just spinning our wheels.

For example, let's say you're trying to get more fit. You could waste time and money and energy researching the best kind of exercise, splash out on a personal trainer, and buy new exercise kit. But what do all those things have in common? They're not actually moving you forward. They only feel like they're important. This is even more the case if you are choosing to plan your all-new exercise regime *instead of* getting out there and moving your body. In the same way, many experienced therapists know that, for some people, therapy itself is a kind of avoidance for dealing with life's issues. So long as you're in therapy for your problems, you don't actually have to go out there and fix them, right?

Get Friends to Hold You Accountable

One of humankind's greatest attributes is our intellect. But it's also true that we can use our brains for astonishing levels of self-deception, avoidance, and denial. If we're not honest with ourselves, we can waste years buying our own lies and giving in to our own excuses and delays. But there's a remedy for this: other people.

Accountability is like an external yardstick that keeps you in check. Deceiving yourself is one thing but convincing someone else is another. Having an accountability buddy keeps you focused, makes sure you're checking in on yourself and your goals, and puts that little bit of positive pressure on you so you don't slacken up. It's really simple: you're far less likely to cheat or procrastinate on your goals if you know someone is watching—all the better if that person is someone whose opinion you value.

"Positive peer pressure" is yet another way we can take conscious control of our lives and use what we have to achieve our goals. If you work toward a goal with a close friend, you can both inspire one another, cheerlead one another on when times are tough and giving up seems tempting, and celebrate with them when you push through and get it done anyway. You are, after all, a social being, and you can use this to your advantage. We all want to belong, we want others to witness our successes, we want to be seen and validated as we struggle with challenges, we want support, and yes, we also want approval and from those we love and for them to celebrate milestones with us.

How to Use This in Your Life Immediately

Friendships are like gold. But not *all* friendships are going to help you become the best you can be. You need to pick your friends wisely and construct a support network that will genuinely inspire, encourage, support, and most importantly, challenge you to become your best self. Choose to surround yourself with people who are diverse and can teach you things. Choose those who have already achieved what you're aiming to achieve so you can use them as models. But also choose people who are a little behind you on the same path because you can derive plenty of meaning and encouragement by being a model and mentor for someone else.

The mark of a true friend is one who is willing and able to help you grow. Many people have close friends who unconsciously don't want them to improve or change. Be very careful about people who love you but will nevertheless sabotage your efforts or keep you as you always have been. Watch out for people who enable rather than support. You need someone you can trust to call you out on your BS!

If you're trying to improve your life, there will be ups, downs, challenges, celebrations, and big changes throughout. A good friend is one that will accompany you on this journey. It's *this* person you should pick for your accountability buddy.

- Sign up for a course or class or challenge together, then gently egg each other on or even introduce a little playful competition.
- Keep your buddy in the loop and share your challenges and successes—you're more likely to stay the course if you're communicating honestly about your experience.

- Ask for help!
- Announce your goals to a select few and ask them directly to help keep you accountable. Check in with them once a week to share progress or ask if you can report back to them as you go. Just knowing they are there and watching you will make you pull up your socks!

Determine What You Can Control

Self-discipline is all about that powerful shift in mindset that comes with realizing that *we are in control of our lives.* There is nobody else to blame, nothing stopping us, and no reason that we can't start right now to improve our situation. However, as with all things in life, balance is important. There is so, so much you can control—but you can't control everything!

Wanting to control things that you actually cannot (and should not) control is not self-discipline but an exercise in futility. More than that, it's a recipe for anxiety and stress. Too much agency, self-restraint, and discipline can start to look like rigid perfectionism. Control freaks are not disciplined or organized—they're simply anxious.

When you find yourself worrying, take a minute to examine the things you actually have control over. Zoom out and be realistic about your true scope of action, your responsibility, and your role in the way that events unfold. Self-discipline will take you far, but there are times in life where what happens is simply not up to you.

But even then, you have options. You can be aware, you can choose, and you can act. You can't prevent a storm from coming but you can prepare for it. You can't control how someone else behaves, but you can control how you react to that.

The key to managing anxiety and worry is to focus on what you can control and worry about those things only. You will find yourself less distracted, less worried, and better able to focus on what actually matters.

Recognize that sometimes, all you can control is your effort and your attitude. But that's a lot! When you invest your energy into the things you can control and pull it away from the things you can't, you'll be much more effective and your anxiety will dissipate. You'll be able to rest knowing that you are doing all that you can—and what else could you do?

How to Use This in Your Life Immediately

The old saying goes, "God, grant me the serenity to accept the things I cannot change, the courage to change the things I cannot accept, and the wisdom to know the difference." So, serenity, courage, and wisdom are needed.

The ancient Stoics had a brilliant method for tackling anxiety, overthinking, and rumination. If you find yourself overcome with worry and anxiety, take it as a sign that you need to pause and have a look at your thoughts, feelings, and behaviors. Take a piece of paper and draw three columns. The first is titled "Things I have zero control over." The second is titled "Things I have a degree of control over." The last is titled "Things I have complete control over."

Now, take a moment to contemplate the issue that's stressing you out, and pick it apart. Let's say you're nervous about an upcoming performance review and are worried about your future job security. Take your time filling out the columns but be as truthful and realistic as possible. You cannot control the performance review that other people give you. You can nudge things this way or that way depending on how you conduct yourself at the end-of-year interview. And you can completely control your overall attitude, response, and future choices. You can control how you frame the situation, whether you blame yourself or others, and what you choose to learn from the situation.

After you've spent some time dissecting the situation (you may need to move things a few times after closer consideration), it's time to act. Remember that you have limited time, resources, energy, and willpower. Remember also that you have values and preferences and goals. Now, with that in mind, how are you going to conduct yourself?

Tear off the first column and throw it away. There's no use spending a second more time on that—why would you when you know it will have zero impact? Next, look at the final column—this is where you can do the most. Once you have acted to fully maximize on those things you can control, you can then look at the middle column and see how you can steer events somewhat. Commit to concrete action. When you're done, put the paper away and tell yourself, "I can relax now. I've done everything I can. The rest is not my business."

Take Ownership and Responsibility

Let's take a closer look at control. No, you don't always have control over things, and when you do, you seldom have complete control.

But what you always do have is ownership and responsibility.

"Owning" something means maturely recognizing that something is, in fact, yours and not someone else's. It's not someone else's job to make you happy or productive, and it's not someone else's fault that you're not. If you feel lazy or angry or undecided or fearful, those feelings belong to you and only you. And that means that you and only you can work to change them. This book is about *self*-discipline, and not discipline. This is about taking responsibility for your own actions. You are not controlled or maneuvered by anyone else or by your environment or events. Yes, events happen and other people choose what they choose, but we are always, always responsible for what we do with our own lives and what we choose.

When you are not responsible for what happens in your life then it means you are a victim. Taking ownership can feel scary if you are used to avoiding or blaming or making excuses, but taking responsibility is actually a kind of freedom, and it connects you to your power in a way that nothing else can.

How to Use This in Your Life Immediately

Taking real responsibility can be lifelong work, but it's something we can constantly hold ourselves accountable to, in every moment.

Firstly, get in the habit of asking, *who does this belong to?*

When you have an emotion, when you speak, when you act, when you think something—who does it belong to? Some people take on too much responsibility and assume that everything is theirs. This question will help you identify that pattern, too. Nobody can *make* you feel or do or say anything, and similarly, you can't *make* anyone else do or say or feel something—not without everyone's permission!

Secondly, notice when you're tempted to complain—complaints often hide blame. If you're unhappy or angry, don't forget to ask what *your role* in the situation is. What are you doing to cause or maintain the problem? Forget about what others should or shouldn't do and look to yourself: what is your scope of action? When you complain, you are disempowering yourself. Stop and immediately ask what action you can take to improve your situation. This will take you out of victim mode and into responsibility.

Another, more subtle way we can fail to take responsibility is to passively wait for better days or assume that someone or something is coming to save us. Watch if you often say "one day" and constantly look forward to the future rather than making the present all it can be. Life is right now. When you assume the good thing is coming later (or already past) you forfeit your own responsibility. Ask instead, "What do I want right now? And what I can I do right now to make that happen?"

Finally, we can all learn to take more responsibility in life in the way we choose to interpret events, where we chose to put our attention, and how we respond to stimuli in our environment—or not. You don't have to take every insult personally. You don't have to agree with other people's interpretations or priorities. If someone projects onto you, you don't have to accept that projection as true. You don't have to be crushed by failure—you can choose to learn from it. When you pursue your own values and seek your own meaning, you are owning your own life. This will give you conviction and courage that will strengthen you more than anything else.

__Practice Gratitude__
Being grateful is not merely a favorable *emotional* state of mind to be in. When you practice gratitude, you are also affecting your cognition, your perception, your problem-solving ability, your creativity, and your resilience. Practicing gratitude is one of those things that looks kind of sweet and nice on the surface, but when practiced

daily, starts to show the full force of its power. It can be a game-changer.

You might not think that gratitude has much to do with self-control, but the two go hand in hand. When you practice gratitude—and also compassion, connectedness, contentment, and even pride—then you are effectively building a store of good feelings and wellbeing that almost inoculate you against future temptations, obstacles, and setbacks.

When you have an ongoing gratitude practice, you are basically cultivating a kind of spiritual immune system that will protect you from disappointment, impatience, fear, and so on. When you can become aware of and relish all the good things in your life, you feel "full"—and this fullness allows you to tackle life's difficulties with a bit more grace.

Consider an example: In the morning, you make yourself a healthy breakfast of oats with blueberries and a delicious cup of coffee. You don't rush and gobble it up though, but pause and savor every bite, truly relishing just how lucky you are to eat such a nice thing in the morning. You leave your house on a positive note, feeling content and satisfied. Later, when you encounter some cake at the office, you're tempted for a moment, but then again, you've already had a nice breakfast and feel good already—what could cake add?

Importantly, nothing's really changed—only your attitude. You have taken the time to notice what is already wonderful in your life and so are less tempted by distractions. You have more self-discipline because you are coming from a place of abundance and contentment, rather than negativity and looking for the worst. Later in the same day, if you hear some bad news, it may sting, but it will probably sting less.

Living your life with gratitude helps you notice the little wins like the bus showing up right on time, a stranger holding the door for you, or the sun shining through your window when you wake up in the morning. Each of these small moments strings together to create a web of well-being that, over time, strengthens your ability to notice the good. And more than that, it helps you spot opportunities or solutions to problems that might have been invisible to your more shut-down, pessimistic brain.

How to Use This in Your Life Immediately

A gratitude journal is a thing of beauty, and it's free and easy to do, right now (Hooray! Let's be thankful for the existence of gratitude journals). Simply open a notebook and get into the daily habit of noting the things you're grateful for. The nice weather. Your cat being a darling. The fact that you got a discount on your burrito. Your back hurt yesterday and it doesn't hurt anymore. You found a penny on the floor. The color pink exists.

Don't limit your spirit of thankfulness to your journal, though. Try to have gratitude glasses on all throughout your day, deliberately looking for all the ways that things are pretty awesome right now. What can you brag about or be proud about? What lucky break have you received? What lovely things in your immediate environment used to give you joy until you got bored and forgot about them? Look for things that are beautiful or funny or comforting. Notice what makes you smile—even tiny things. Say thank you—out loud or just internally—and thank even the items in your house as you use them. Isn't it nice that you have your faithful coffee mug, always there for you? Thanks coffee mug.

Don't just do lip service; really cultivate the feeling of gratitude. Pause and let that feeling of thankfulness and contentment settle in. Feel blessed. Soak it up and imagine yourself storing up those good vibes to carry into the rest of your life.

Believe in Willpower

Finally, let's look at one last attitude that predicts and supports your success on the path to your goals: self-belief. This is in fact scientifically proven: *if you believe you can do it and use self-discipline, then it will be true.* This is great news for you, since in reading this book, at least part of you must believe that it's possible to grow your willpower and use it to better your life.

Willpower, it seems, is not quite enough on its own. Rather, what's effective seems to be your accompanying set of beliefs, interpretations, and expectations when it comes to willpower.

What is willpower, really? It's simply the ability to put off instant gratification and deliberately, consciously choose to act toward your long term-goals instead. This ability has been shown to predict better school performance, greater self-confidence, lower likelihood of substance abuse or addiction problems, better financial health, and greatly improved physical and mental health, too. With self-discipline, you develop the patience, commitment, and consistency needed to achieve the things that really matter.

But digging deeper, this self-discipline must come from an abiding belief that you can do in fact something to better your situation. You need to truly believe that you are in control, that change is possible, and that you can achieve that change with consistent self-discipline action. The action absolutely matters, but that action is informed by *belief*.

How strong is your will, really? How able are you to bring about your wishes, desires and plans through effort and action alone? Whatever your answer is, then *that* is itself the size of your willpower. If you say, "I don't think I have much willpower" then how could you ever act to achieve your will? But if you say, "I have my convictions, and I believe I can do it, in fact I *know* I can . . ." then you already have a vastly greater chance of actually succeeding than the other person. Even if you and the other person possess equal resources, opportunities and abilities. That's a big deal.

How to use this in your life immediately

Having self-belief may come across as one of those cheesy things people work on in self-help books, but the fact is that there is an almost magical ability of your body and mind to follow through on what your conscious has already decided is the case. It's easy to start fostering this belief in yourself.

In 2018, Michael Inzlicht, a University of Toronto psychologist, asked participants to rate themselves according to how self-disciplined they were. It turns out, those who rated themselves highly were also found to actually have happier lives, better relationships and so on. The interesting thing is that independent tests of these people's willpower showed that they didn't in fact possess any special abilities others didn't—they just *believed* they did. But that belief mattered.

Inzlicht and other researchers like him have since discovered that people who do well in this area are not more self-disciplined exactly, but they genuinely do enjoy the habits that are good for them, and seem to have a more positive view on their power to resist temptation. Developing this for yourself is two-fold. You need to a) develop better habits and learn useful techniques for managing temptation and sticking to good habits but also b) you need to believe that this is possible, and that you personally can do it with effort.

If you find yourself lacking in this area, the irony is that simply having a little faith in yourself will start to shift things for you! As we've seen, gratitude, responsibility, honesty and allowing others to hold you accountable are great ways to improve your life, but there's also a lot to be said for simply believing in yourself. Whatever your weaknesses are, whatever your obstacles, hold onto the idea that **it can change**, and you can change it. It's this attitude that will most empower you. Every morning, wake up and say to yourself, "I can do this." Your "this" will change day to day, but so long as you have self-belief, you will have a much greater chance of achieving it, whatever "this" is.

Summary:

- Your success is determined by your attitude. Get real and honest with yourself and remove those things in life that seem like they're making you productive but are actually just wasting your time. Keep asking, "Does this move me forward?"
- Use positive peer pressure to keep you accountable to your commitments. Rope in friends to witness your achievements, support you, and inspire you when you're having trouble.
- Have a healthy attitude toward control—though there are things in life we never have control over, we are always in charge of our own reactions and actions. Try the Stoic exercise to help you identify what you can change, what you can't, and practice the wisdom it takes to know the difference.

- Self-disciplined people know that their success in life is their own responsibility, and they own it. They don't blame others, complain, or wait for permission. They embrace the freedom of responsibility.
- A regular gratitude practice keeps you in a positive frame of mind, makes you more resilient, more creative, and better able to control yourself. Find things to be thankful for every single day, and fill yourself up with good feelings that make self-discipline easier.
- Finally, if you believe you can do it, you can. Self-belief is a powerful predictor of success, so have a little faith in yourself!

Chapter 5: Stay Mindful

Meditate to Activate

No book on self-discipline and productivity would be complete without a mention of mindfulness. By now, almost everyone knows that meditation is a powerful way to combat stress, cultivate greater wellbeing and develop greater self-awareness. There's no doubt that regular meditation connects us to our spirituality, helps us tune into our values, gives us time and space to experience gratitude, and improves body awareness. Something you may not be aware of, though, is meditation's capacity to help you strengthen your self-control.

The reason is that meditation and mindfulness practices have been shown via neuroimaging studies to increase neural activation and boost connectivity in those parts of the brain we know are related to self-regulation. A 2014 study in the *Annals of the New York Academy of Sciences* strongly suggests that meditation is not just great for stress and mental wellbeing, but for self-discipline. If you've ever meditated for any length of time, you can probably guess why. The task of the meditator is essentially one of quiet self-regulation and control. So far in this book we've spoken about becoming aware of patterns and the source of behaviors, and of pausing to take the time to consciously choose differently. This awareness and consciousness are exactly what is being developed when we meditate.

Meditation trains us to be more aware and less emotionally reactive. Thus, we are aware of our emotions *as emotions*, and are conscious and awake enough to choose how we react, rather than getting carried away with distraction, addiction, fear, and laziness.

Meditation requires discipline, but discipline is also fostered with the ongoing practice of meditation. When we sit down to meditate, day after day, no matter what, we strengthen our resolve and learn habits that translate into every area of life. We gain perspective, practice being consistent, and notice the rising and falling of challenges, excitement, distractions. We watch them arise and watch them pass. Our commitment is like a rock in the stream—they flow around and past us.

How to Use This in Your Life Immediately

People can be intimidated by meditation or view it as a boring, complicated slog. It isn't. It's very, very simple:

Step 1: Have a little faith that learning anything new takes patience and a little motivation.

Step 2: Set your intention. Remember that small steps maintained consistently are more valuable than quantum leaps. For example, decide that you will meditate for a minimum of five minutes every single day, rain or shine.

Step 3: Follow through. When you encounter an obstacle, smile and make friends with it. Watch yourself pushing past it. Practice self-compassion—you don't need to be perfect, just pitch up, be kind to yourself, and be aware. Notice that over time, you *are* improving. Even if all you do one day is sit down and fight with yourself in your head for ten minutes, fine. Just become aware of that. And the next day, sit down again and become aware again. Sometimes, the biggest strides made in your practice are not during your time spent mediating, but the time *between* sessions.

That said, it's worth making sure that you're not undermining your meditation efforts during the rest of your day. Do your best to stay mindful *always*, not just when you're meditating. Pay attention to what's going on in your body, in your mind, and in your environment. Pause, take a deep breath and become aware of your options. This alone will build up grey matter in your brain's self-regulation centers. Notice how your diet, sleep habits, and consumption of mind-altering substances (yes, that includes caffeine, alcohol, and over-the-counter medications!) affects your state of mind, and commit to reducing them. Finally, any type of meditation can be beneficial, but simple breathing meditations or guided forms may be best for beginners.

Keep Calm, Keep Mindful

Meditation is a more formalized way to practice being mindful, aware and conscious in each moment. A daily meditation practice will definitely bring more peace and relaxation into your life, but you don't need to do formal meditation practices to bring more mindfulness and calm into your life. It's a mistake to think that a hectic, reactive, and negative lifestyle can be cancelled out with just twenty minutes sitting on a cushion! In other words, it's better to practice stillness and awareness as *a way of life* rather than a discrete event you do now and then.

When you are calm, quiet and centered, you are incredibly powerful. If you can pause and open a space of awareness for yourself in the moment, then you give yourself access to possibilities. You become aware of your choices and can make those choices consciously. You are les emotionally reactive, less stressed, less rushed, and far more likely to tune into your values and principles, as well as your long-term goals and commitments.

Being calm and quiet is not just something that feels nice, or something we do to counteract stress. Learning to regularly quieten down our nervous system actually sets the stage for discipline, mindfulness and intelligent choices. We are able to be mentally, emotion ally and physically resilient. Self-discipline and being cool, calm and collected go hand in hand.

How to Use This in Your Life Immediately

What does this actually look like, day to day?

If you practice meditation regularly, you'll strengthen that muscle that allows you to stop in the middle of an emotionally charged moment and say, "Wait a second. What am I feeling right now? What's going on?" If you're aware of yourself becoming stressed, unhappy, over-tired, or angry, then you can push the pause button. Create a little bit of space for yourself. Imagine it as opening a small window in your awareness for some fresh air.

Now, take some deep belly breaths, focusing on making the exhale longer. This will regulate your central nervous system and signal to your body that it's time to relax. From this state, you can let your higher, conscious mind take action according to what actually matters to you.

Try to notice what you're feeling, body and mind. Try to put a word to your emotion and notice what your body is doing. No judgment—just awareness. Tell yourself that these feelings are transient and will pass.

If you're really stressed or alarmed, sometimes the best thing you can do is engage in physical activity. Go for a run or long walk or do something like deep clean your kitchen. This releases tension and channels emotions into energy and action. Alternatively, you could ask your body what it needs and find you feel better after listening to some music, taking a break, or doing something that makes you feel good. A little bit of fresh air, a deep stretch to release tension from slouching, or a brief mindfulness exercise can center and ground you.

If you notice yourself getting carried away with thoughts, it may help to write them down. This slows anxious rumination (try the Stoic activity from above) and helps you narrow down what's bothering you. You'll find that simply dumping thoughts somewhere "out there" in the world brings clarity and a sense of calm.

It can be hard to remain calm if you have a high-pressure job or are dealing with life challenges. But remember, you can always pause to take a breath, become aware of where you are, and consciously take action in the direction *you* choose. Don't rush. If necessary, ask people for more time or tell them you'll get back to them. Set boundaries. A calmer life for many people means more delegation and dropping clutter, literal or metaphorical, from their lives.

Drop the Ego

We don't meditate to earn accolades, or compete with others, or brag. Meditation and mindfulness are ways to become more deeply and clearly acquainted with the present moment. When we meditate, our mental churnings, our personal myths and narratives, our ruminations and excuses and internal dramas—all of these are set aside so we can access still, calm consciousness, right now. This means that ego doesn't play a role.

Many people seek personal development and strive to be more productive and successful primarily as an ego exercise. Now, "ego" doesn't just mean that you're arrogant and self-centered—it's broader than that, and denotes any state of mind where you are hung up on your own sense of personal identity and self. A person who thinks too highly of themselves and is unable to hear criticism has let their ego take over. But on the other hand, someone who is stubbornly attached to an image of themselves as a loser, and who cannot hear praise or risk trying something new—they have an ego problem, too.

We can think of the ego as a veil between who you think you are and who you really are. It's like a mask we wear as we move around the world and interact with others. We *need* an ego—it's like a vehicle. But it's a question of being mindful of the role our ego is playing. There's no need to "kill" the ego or imagine that we need to be selfless monks and nuns with zero personal identity!

Let's put all of this into the context of self-discipline. Can your ego get in the way of you being your most productive, most effective and most determined self? Absolutely.

Firstly, your ego can make it hard for you to take risks or trying something new, because you're afraid of what others might think. A big ego can make you avoid being a beginner, asking for help, admitting mistakes, or looking a little silly while you're learning something new. As a result, your ego remains intact but you learn nothing!

The go can also trap us in all our old stories and beliefs. The ego is like a fixed role you play; if you're constantly thinking, "Oh no, my character could never do *that*," then you are limiting and even undermining yourself. To protect your ego, you could avoid new or challenging situations, ignore valuable criticism and feedback, or simply fail to grow and evolve because something doesn't seem like it fits who you are now.

How to Use This in Your Life Immediately

Keeping a toxic ego in check is not difficult—it's something we can do every day, if we only remain mindful:

- Keep your attention on the process and not the outcome. It's all that you can really control anyway, and

focusing on it will prevent you getting distracted by rewards, praise, and so on.
- Always consider yourself a beginner. Get comfortable saying "I don't know." Any time you learn something new, there's something else beyond the horizon. Stay humble and resist the urge to be the expert who has it all figured out. Certainty is stagnation!
- Tell yourself that failing or making mistakes doesn't define you—and that means ultra-success doesn't either. Use an internal measure of your own self-worth, that isn't vulnerable to what shifts and changes externally. This means you need to know yourself on a deep level, and work with a purpose.
- Promise yourself to give up the habit of comparison. While you're at it, cut short any desire to gossip or complain.
- Get out of your own head. Regularly engage with people who have different perspectives, welcome diversity of thought, and keep

- humble by reminding yourself of the bigger picture you're a part of.
- Dedicate yourself to your *purpose*—that thing you would do even if nobody ever recognized or praised it, that thing that is above your own pride and satisfaction.
- Realize that you are not entitled to anything. At the same time, know that you are allowed to choose your own values, and stick with them, regardless of what others say.

Know the Difference Between Suffering and Pain

The Buddhists knew a lot about self-discipline, non-reactivity, and inner calm. One brilliant lesson we can borrow from this philosophy is the attitude toward pain and suffering—which are not the same thing!

In life, pain is inevitable, but suffering is optional.

What does this mean? We all live in flawed physical bodies that will eventually decay and perish. We all live in a world where things are transient, and where loss is a given. So, we experience pain. People we love die. Accidents happen. We get ill, we break something, we stub our toes. This is all pain—and it's a normal and natural part of life.

However, suffering is one step further. Suffering is our mind's attachment to pain. It's all the stories and narratives we weave around pain. Self-pity, denial, worry, regret, indignation, complaining . . . all of these things are separate from the original pain. These are sometimes called "second darts." If you were shot with a dart, it would hurt like hell. This is the first dart. But if you then pulled the dart out and spent the next three days raging against the person who threw the dart, that would be a "second dart." That would be a kind of pain and unhappiness that was purely optional. So, if you tell yourself a story like, "That pain *should not* have happened, and I'm really mad now, and I won't let it go . . ." you are creating suffering for yourself—and sometimes the suffering is much worse than the pain!

So, the way you think about pain matters. When you are mindful, you can be aware of the difference, and notice whether you are actively choosing to suffer. Remember that you cannot change the fact of pain. In fact, pain is useful for the body, and alerts us to danger, inspiring us to beneficial action. Pain is inevitable, but suffering is not. The goal is not to live a painless life. The goal is to stop creating unnecessary and avoidable suffering for yourself. To stop blaming others, making excuses, projecting onto others, bargaining, condemning, judging, or engaging in negative self-talk that does nothing to improve the situation.

What should our attitude to pain be? We can sit with it, and let it pass. We don't have to like it, but there's no reason to wrestle with it. There's no point arguing with it.

And our attitude to suffering? Well, we need to remember that suffering is something that we have control over. Let's turn our attention away from pain (which, after all, we can't do anything about) and onto suffering [which we can].

How to use this in your life immediately

Yes, we want to "mind our mood" and get into our conscious, rational decision-making mind. But we also don't want to try and *get rid* of bad feelings, push them away, diminish them, or judge them. The first step is awareness, and closely on its heels is acceptance. If it hurts, fine. Just be with that. The first step is to accept that we are in pain and be aware of our suffering.

Without any need to judge, interpret, fix or deny, simply sit with the pain that's there. Be curious about it. Be still and see what it is, without trying to run away, grab hold of it, or shove it out of awareness. Take lots of deep breaths and a little time—can you discern the difference between pure, simple pain right now and suffering, i.e., your attachment and stories surrounding that pain? Remember, you're just in an exploratory frame of mind, you're not diagnosing or assessing or making stories.

When a story comes up (for example, "I love my work so if I'm unmotivated, it means I'm weak somehow" or "This always happens . . ."), just notice it. Don't judge this, either. Just bring awareness to it and see how these stories fit into your ego identity. Gradually, both the suffering and the pain do what they do when you're not holding onto them—they pass.

Get Acquainted with Your Weaknesses

Staying mindful and conscious of what's going on in body and mind is potent way of staying on top of self-discipline simply because the more you know, the better prepared you can be. As we saw in an earlier chapter, a big part of managing temptations is being aware of what triggers you to cheat or stray in the first place, and then avoiding those things you know will distract or derail you. This only works, of course, if you actually have real insight into how you tick. If we can drop our egos enough to be honest about our weak points, we can pre-empt any temptations or challenges and act to avoid them before they trip us up.

Our mindfulness tips so far have understandably focused on being present in the moment, but sometimes being more mindful means understanding how you will act *in the future*, and then adjusting accordingly. Knowledge is power, as they say, and *self*-knowledge is *self*-power!

Be proactive. Why put yourself in the position of having to fend of temptation in the moment when you can avoid it hours or days before? If you know you need to run a 5K this Saturday but your friend is having a barbeque on Friday night, it might be best to skip it. That single decision, powered by knowledge of your weaknesses and common-sense about how events are likely to unfold, saves you from having to wrestle with yourself later on. If you know that having snack food in the pantry leads you to go on a binge and eat it all, don't keep food in the pantry.

It's a very empowering perspective to take: we all have weaknesses, yes, but we also possess the tools to fight back against these demons. All that's needed is honest self-awareness of where you are right now, and an intelligent strategy for working around your blind spots.

How to Use This in Your Life Immediately

Hooray! It's list time again. Make two lists—on one list write down all the value you bring to the world. Think of those things that come easy to you, your skills and passions. Think of those things that you can do for hours and never procrastinate on. The other list contains your weaknesses. Don't beat yourself up though, this is just about those things that are challenging right now for you, those things you're not comfortable or familiar with, or those things that you've struggled with in the past.

Bringing self-awareness to both these aspects helps because it can guide your action:

For your <u>strengths</u>, constantly ask how you can leverage what you're already good at and make the best use of your natural talents and passions. Look at the things on your list and ask if you have enough opportunity to enjoy, benefit from or express these aspects.

For your <u>weaknesses</u>, constantly ask what more you need to do to develop (again, this best done with as little ego as possible!). For some weaknesses, you may never "fix" them, but you can definitely work around them, pre-empt them or mitigate them.

Even better if you can use your strengths to almost bootstrap improvement with your weaknesses—i.e., how can you use your talents to balance, offset, or improve on those less developed parts of yourself?

Remember to be honest about your strengths and don't think that your weaknesses are a shortcoming—in fact, they are your teachers and will show you the areas where you have most to gain if you invest in them.

Takeaways:

- Being mindful and meditating are not just ways to reduce stress and improve wellbeing; they're techniques to strengthen self-awareness, lower reactivity and improve self-discipline. When you meditate, you activate the parts of your brain responsible for self-control, strengthening those neural connections.
- Meditation is not just a discrete activity but a way of life. Find ways to become aware throughout the day and use these feelings of calm control and mindfulness to reconnect to your self-discipline. Pause, become aware of what's going on inside you and outside you in your

environment, and notice your thoughts and feelings without judgment or interpretation.
- A major stumbling block for those wanting to develop better self-discipline and improve their lives as letting their ego get in the way. The ego is a mask; it's not the real you. Regularly remind yourself of the process, not the outcome and be okay with being a beginner or being wrong. Stop playing a role and encounter the moment as it is—no comparisons, appraisals, or judgments.
- On your self-discipline journey, you'll encounter pain, which is inevitable. But suffering (i.e., the way we react to pain) is avoidable. Blame, personal narratives, regret, self-hate, doubt, anxiety etc. are all optional reactions. Try not to add "second darts" when life deals you a bad hand. With awareness and calm, compassionate acceptance, we can allow both pain and suffering to pass.
- Knowledge is power, and self-knowledge is self-power. If you know your strengths and weaknesses, you can consciously work around your blind spots while maximizing on your good attributes. Don't see your flaws as

shortcomings, but instead learn what you can from them and focus on the good.

Chapter 6: Get Organized with Your Time

Put the Big Rocks in First

Time management is all about understanding what your priorities are, so that you can focus on those *first*. Though this makes a lot of intuitive sense, the fact is that most of us tend to delay or dawdle on the things that are actually most important to us, choosing instead to focus on tasks that simply don't add anything to the bigger picture.

In the '80s, self-help author and productivity guru Steven Covey was the first to popularize the concept of "eating the frog" first thing in the morning. Basically, this means doing the most important thing (or else the most challenging or demanding thing) first in the morning. The idea is that if you make this a temporal priority, you will not give yourself the chance to get distracted or tempted by other unimportant information. You won't get sidetracked by all those little tasks that seem like they're important, but actually don't move you forward one inch on your path.

Remember, you are dealing with several limited resources: time, willpower, and energy . . . not to mention opportunities. If you want to be an effective human being and accomplish your dreams, not just one day but as *soon as possible*, then you need to maximize on the resources you have. You have no choice but to be ruthless in cutting away distraction, temptation and irrelevant information.

Think of "big rocks" as your priorities. These are the goals, actions or events that carry the most significance or impact. Here's the analogy: imagine a big glass jar. Your goal is to fill it up as much as possible. If you fill it with little rocks first, it's far harder to then find space for a big rock. But if you put your big rocks in first, then there's always a few corners to squeeze in a few small rocks, if you need to.

The glass jar is fixed in size and represents your limited resources. The big rocks are your priorities, and the little rocks are all those daily tasks that can clutter up your schedule and make you feel "bust"—without actually being productive. Typically, people lose productivity because they have no idea what their big rocks are, they have too many (which is almost the same as having none), or they cannot pull themselves away from the trifling, mindless "small rock" tasks that waste their time and energy.

Having a priority means that certain things necessarily go on the back burner. In fact, you'll have to say no to *most* things. This takes discipline—but it also encourages discipline. If it's 10 a.m. and you've already done your most effective and impactful work for the day, imagine how good you'd feel. You'd find room in the rest of your day to do all those trifling tasks, but they'd have their proper place—*after* you'd done the truly important thing.

How to Use This in Your Life Immediately

The first step is to obviously identify your big rocks. To do this, first get an idea of all the tasks you typically occupy yourself with and then group them according to these categories:

- Not urgent and not important (water)
- Urgent but not important (gravel and sand)
- Important but not urgent (small stones)
- Urgent and important (big rocks)

Urgent and important tasks are done first, always. Important but not urgent tasks are done next, *before* those things that are urgent but not important. Finally, tasks that are not urgent or important can be delegated, ignored or pushed down the list to when you have a free moment, if you want to. Don't be heroic and try to do *everything*—this is not the path to productivity. If you don't put the big rocks in first, believe me, you will not be able to put them in later.

Keep in mind that there's no point arguing with the resources you have available—the glass jar is as big as it is, and that's that. Your productivity will come from having the self-discipline to prioritize and organize your schedule to reflect the big rocks. The gravel and rocks and sand tend to sort themselves out one way or another. Focus on looking at your schedule and making sure the big rocks are getting first place in your day.

Time Management According to Your Unique Rhythms

Of course, this is assuming that the morning is actually your most productive time of day. Your "biological prime time" may in fact be a completely different time of day. Each of us has our own innate body rhythms and our energy, productivity and creativity rise and fall in waves over a twenty-four-hour period. We need to carefully identify when our unique periods of peak productivity and energy fall. This way, we can schedule our time accordingly, making the most of our time and energy. Think of it this way: if you practice a little self-discipline at first and identify your golden work periods, then in essence you need *less* self-discipline overall because you'll be moving with your natural flows rather than against them.

How to Use This in Your Life Immediately

Again: self-knowledge is power here. To begin, take a week or two where you simply stay in observation mode and watch to see what your normal rhythms are like. Make no assumptions. Keep a journal where you note down, in hourly increments, your energy levels on a scale of one to ten. You could choose a single metric, i.e., how much work you tend to get done, or break it down into several measures, for example, energy, creativity, optimism, etc. The more data you gather the better, so take your time and look for patterns. Don't presume that you'll be more energetic in the morning, and try not to interfere with your natural cycles by skimping on sleep or using stimulants or depressants (caffeine and alcohol are the biggest culprits, respectively).

Once you've gathered some information about how your energy and productivity flows, take a moment to compile it and represent it visually. Some people literally draw a graph showing shifting energy patterns over twenty-four hours. Now, on the one hand you have your natural flow of energy, and on the other, you can have your daily schedule and routine. Your goal is to match and align these two as far as possible without causing too much disruption to your existing routine.

Doing this work takes discipline, but if done correctly, you are actually giving yourself less work to do; you won't be "swimming upstream" energy-wise and will get more done without having to force or push through energy slumps. Sometimes, self-discipline is less about white-knuckling your way through things day after day, and instead working smart to pre-empt, plan, and strategize once so that every day flows more smoothly without as much conscious effort.

Remember your big rocks? Those should be aligned with your peak energy periods. Save the low-skilled, mundane work for when you're feeling less creative and optimistic. When you are naturally feeling restful and quiet, plan breaks and naps so you get the most from your body's ability to recharge. For example, you may identify a golden period of three hours every morning from around 10:30 to 13:30. Eat your frogs during this time. Then, get stuck into the other less important tasks. By the time it's evening, and your energy and enthusiasm is waning, do things like clean, cook, socialize, read, exercise, meditate, and so on.

Bear in mind that you will likely discover *different* peaks throughout your day—for example you may feel mentally most alive in the morning, physically strongest in the early afternoon and most able to solve problems and dream of creative solutions in the early evening. Plan accordingly.

<u>The Power of a Countdown</u>
Isn't it a wonderful thing, to know that you always, *always* have the power to change your focus and your mood? No matter what has come before, you always possess the ability to stop, become aware and decide how you want to express your own personal power. Some people find it easy to cultivate a great attitude throughout the day and stay mindful and positive pretty easily. However, things go haywire when some especially strong emotion comes along, and they feel unable to "snap" out of it.

Are you someone who can get swallowed up by an anxiety spiral that comes out of nowhere? Do you have a bad temper and find yourself losing your cool so quickly that you lash out before you even know what's happening? Do you find yourself getting swept away quickly by negative self-talk that completely ruins your mood in the space of a few minutes? You might like to try a few techniques for rapidly gaining control of yourself again, *in the moment*. Sometimes, we just need a little push, a quick distraction, or a psychological jolt to break us out of negative old patterns and get our forward momentum going again.

How to Use This in Your Life Immediately

Here are some ways to snap yourself back onto the path and quickly pull yourself out of negative or distracting loops. Now, these techniques themselves won't address any underlying problems, but they will allow you to quickly come to a calmer, more rationally frame of mind where deeper analysis and action is possible.

One method is to use a countdown. Let's say you're feeling really lazy and unmotivated. Simply count down from ten, and then act. Count down, then get up off the sofa and start, or pick up your pen or book. Sounds simple, but this is a powerful psychological trick that cuts through excuses and stories and gets you in the right frame of mind.

On the other hand, if anxiety is your problem, recognize that you're not a slave to it and can take action to reduce worried feelings. One way is the 5, 4, 3, 2, 1 technique: take a few deep breaths, then notice your environment. Find five things you can see, four things you can hear, three things you can touch, two things you can smell, and one thing you can taste. This grounding technique stills your mind and brings your attention not where it matters: the present. Then, carry on (perhaps with a countdown!). Another way to manage anxiety is to literally burn it off. Do vigorous exercise, which will flood your body with endorphins and calm you, as well as put you in an active, proactive frame of mind.

If anger is something that threatens to derail your disciplined productivity, then a countdown can help as well—stop, take a deep breath, and count down from ten before you do or say anything else. You might like to step outside for a moment, be in nature, stretch your muscles, distract yourself, listen to some music or generally put yourself in a brief time out until your anger subsides. When you're feeling more level-headed, don't just go back into things—ask if there is an *appropriate action* that your anger is pointing toward.

The key to snapping out of strong emotions or tempting loops is to get back into the present. Do this by pausing, becoming aware, and getting in touch with your five senses. All you need to do is create a single moment of clarity. Then, in that moment, choose the right thing. Count down to ten. Carry on.

Avoid Procrastination—Methods that Work

I'm going to let you in on a little secret: dealing with procrastination is pretty easy. There's a reason we've waited this long to delve into procrastination—it's because once you master self-discipline more generally, create a healthy lifestyle, and get your attitude right, you will not have to wrestle with procrastination. Because it simply won't happen all that often. *Avoiding* procrastination is infinitely better than trying to battle it once it's well underway.

Once embedded, procrastination can indeed wreak havoc on your dreams, your decision making and your self-esteem. People who are self-disciplined don't possess any magical power to remain motivated at all times or somehow force themselves to get to work when they feel lazy. Rather, they *understand* motivation and why it wanes sometimes, and they know how to work with and around those challenges when they emerge.

If you have clearly outlined your goals, organized yourself by making a realistic schedule, and addressed any resistant around those goals, half the work is done. With a positive attitude, healthy lifestyle, and enough appropriate rewards and breaks, you should be able to cut procrastination down in your life. Yes, all of us feel a little lazy now and then, but if everything else in your life is well-aligned, you can take the existence of procrastination as a helpful sign that you still have work to do on your organization, your mindset, your goals, your lifestyle or all of these.

Procrastination is a reinforcing and self-amplifying cycle, and once it starts it can be difficult to stop. But if it doesn't get the chance to start, it's far easier to avoid and prevent. Be on the lookout for early signs and step in quickly, without judgment. Here are two main ways to make sure you're never really letting procrastination get its foot in the door, or else minimizing its impact once it's started.

How to Use This in Your Life Immediately

The first way is to try and understand what's happening and why. Ordinarily we rely on our self-control and motivation to get us to do what we need to. If this process isn't working, look closely at where and why it's not.

Is there something actively demotivating you?

Is there something practical hindering your action?

There can be a million different reasons we procrastinate—lack of energy, a perfectionist attitude, poor planning and organization, feeling overwhelmed or out of our depth, unconsciously not wanting to do the task at all, low self-esteem, poorly defined goals, lack of a meaningful reward or incentive, fear of positive or negative outcomes, depression—which one is behind your procrastination? Yes, it could be pure laziness. But there also may be something more serious that you need to address.

In this book, we've looked at ways to improve your raw self-control and self-discipline, but if your procrastination stems from another issue, then that will need to be resolved if you hope to find productivity and forward movement again.

Once you have honestly identified the reason for your procrastination, you can make meaningful steps toward fixing the issue. But if you're procrastinating for a more complex reason, trying to develop better self-discipline may only act as a temporary Band-Aid.

If, however, the reason for your procrastination is pretty simple, then so should your strategies. The best thing for beating procrastination? Restore your momentum at any cost. Yes, we said that we should tackle our big rocks first. But if you're feeling stuck and uninspired, do the opposite—break the task down into tiny chunks and do one—just one—to get yourself moving again. Then give yourself a reward.

Often, procrastination is just our brains convincing us that doing the task is impossible or unpleasant. Do *anything* you can to prove yourself wrong.

Cut Your To-Do List in Half
It's kind of ironic: when you picture someone who is "productive," you imagine them being super busy and having crammed full schedules. The truth is that the world's most productive people are actually the most self-disciplined and have learned to be really careful about what they *don't do*. When you cut your to-do list down, you are not doing less. You are doing **more**.

It's far better to do a few things well than to rush and half-heartedly complete many insignificant things. It comes down to focus, values and your true goals. Self-discipline is what allows you to keep on tuning out the noise and refocus in on what actually matters—either the goal itself or the tasks that will get you closer to it.

Again, a sign of poor time and resource management is if you feel you are constantly draining your willpower and time on beating away distractions and temptations. You will be far happier if you design your entire life and daily routine in such a way that you simply don't encounter these things all that often.

Depending on the nature of the work you're trying to do, your work style and your constraints, it might actually make more sense for you to create a don't-do list than a to-do list. This pulls your focus onto what matters and helps you get things done. It also means you save yourself that precious mental bandwidth—after all, clutter in your schedule can be organizational, but we can also be weighed down and distracted by psychological baggage, worries and other ways to waste time.

You don't need to create a don't-do list to make this principle work, however. You can start every day by looking at what you've planned for yourself and then ask, "what is no longer relevant here? What can I delete, delegate or rework?" No, it's not an excuse to procrastinate, but rather trim down things so you're constantly working on the most essential tasks. It's okay to update your priorities. It's okay to ditch certain tasks you planned earlier because things are now different. And it's okay to ignore something without guilt if you decide it's just not super relevant. Less is more.

There are a few clues that you need to prune down your to-do list—or at least update the way you write your lists. If you notice that you are consistently leaving a huge number of items on the list incomplete, that's a sign you've allocated yourself too much to do. Continuing to create long lists that you never fully complete just wastes time, not to mention having those unticked items just makes you feel bad. You are not actually giving yourself the opportunity to ask how you can actually get those things done, rather than just sticking with a list technique that doesn't actually work for you. If your to-do list makes you feel overwhelmed or like you want to procrastinate, that's a bad sign too, as is feeling as though you're being rule dover by this list.

How to Use This in Your Life Immediately

When it comes down to it, there are only a limited number of actions you can take on any one task:

- You can **DO** it yourself, right now.
- You can **DELEGATE** it.
- You can **DEFER** it for later.
- You can **FILE** it away to keep.
- You can **DELETE** it and never think about it again.

What you want to avoid is filling up your life and your to-do list with actions or tasks that are none of the above, i.e., mindlessly stressing about something without doing anything about it, or moving a piece of paper from one place to another.

How do you decide what to do with the various tasks you encounter in your day? As above, you ask whether they are

a) Important or
b) urgent

Important and urgent: do it or delegate it.

Important but not urgent: defer it or file it.

Urgent but not important: defer, delegate or delete.

Not important and not urgent: delegate or delete.

Once you've made your decision, act and don't second guess yourself. Don't just make a list and go; take the time to compile something that works. For most of us, this means making it fifty percent smaller at least!

Seek Patterns—and Change Them

In earlier chapters, we talked about understanding and working with unique physiological rhythms, as well as understanding the form of the procrastination cycle as well as how and why temptation occurs, again and again, in the same way. These are patterns. Often, we become aware of isolated behaviors that we want to change, but these behaviors are actually part of a wider pattern that repeats throughout life. With some of the mindfulness and meditation techniques we've discussed, and by bringing more conscious awareness to what we're doing and why, we can start to see our triggers, our default mindsets, our ingrained reactions. But the idea is simple: if you can observe and understand these patterns, you have a chance of changing them.

Patterns are habits that have bedded down deeply into our personalities, self-concept and mindset. But they can change! We can understand our life as a great, interconnected *system*, and our behaviors and thoughts as *processes*. This gives us insight into the bigger picture. So far we've looked at small pixels of what makes the picture of "self-discipline" but I'm sure you're getting a sense of the bigger system at play in a self-disciplined, productive and successful life.

Now, having patterns you'd rather not have (such as ongoing negative self-talk or repeating relationship issues or the same health concerns happening over and over) is normal. We all have them. But we can choose to be

a) mindful
b) honest and
c) proactive

to change these patterns. We can use the insight that we're following a pattern as a clue that helps teach us to become better. Having a weakness or blind spot isn't necessarily a problem, if you are actively, consciously and honestly working around it while simultaneously playing to your strengths.

How to Use This in Your Life Immediately

As usual, it starts with awareness. Found yourself procrastinating one again or doing something you know will hurt your future self? Great. Pause and become aware. Slow down and pick apar the process which led to the result you're seeing. What triggered it? What was the context? How did you feel? What actions or thoughts or feelings immediately preceded it? What was the outcome? How does this compare to times in the past where it's happened? As you consider this, you're gradually arriving at the answer to the question—*can you see a pattern*? Hey, sometimes there's a one-off event that doesn't mean anything. But look with open eyes and see if you can find repetition, habit and mindlessness. Sometimes, what looks like chaos and randomness is actually just a bigger pattern we haven't yet recognized. If you feel like you're reliving the same scene, the same drama, the same relationship over and over—it's a clue that it's time to grow and change.

Find the logic of what's happening. See yourself a being who is organizing their lives and their selves . . . what are the rules of this organization? What function is this pattern currently serving? You could also share your insights with trusted others, since other people are often good at spotting our patterns before we do.

To start gaining insight into your own patterns, you need to do only a few simple (but not easy) things:

- Pay attention!
- Become aware and see the pattern as clearly as possible
- Consciously commit to breaking out of it with action

So, for a simple example, you might notice that your willpower disappears every time you hang out with certain people, you're triggered into a series of behaviors that ends with you behaving in ways you don't want to. You work backward and decide to chance the pattern, maybe a little (you meet them in a different environment), maybe a lot (you stop meeting them at all).

Takeaways:

- Willpower is a limited resource but so is time. Self-discipline requires conscious control over how we spend our time. Follow Stephen Covey's advice and "put the big rocks first"—the less important tasks of life can be squeezed in later. Start the day with your priorities.
- Not everyone will follow the same sleep/wakefulness cycles; it's up to you to understand your own rhythms and work with them. Identify your peak energy periods and schedule your most important or demanding tasks for this time. You need less self-discipline if you're working with your natural motivational flow.
- A great way to break out of inaction or overcome strong derailing emotions is to count down from ten and then just force yourself to act. Anxiety can be tackled by becoming aware of the present moment on all five senses. Anger can be managed by hitting the pause button, breathing deeply, and having a time out.

- Procrastination can be a sign that your organization, goals or mindset are not where they should be, but all of us procrastinate out of laziness from time to time. Fix the problem by restoring momentum as soon as you can. Get started with just the tiniest task first or promise yourself you'll do just five minutes. If your procrastination comes from deeper issues, you need to tackle these first.
- A to-do list can help focus you, but if you're a chronic over-doer, a don't-do list may be more appropriate. Look at every item on your list and ask whether it is urgent and important. Tasks that are neither can be ignored or delegated, tasks that are both should be prioritized.
- Finally, become adept at noticing your own behavioral patterns. Be mindful, honest and proactive in recognizing where you're repeating the same patterns over and over. Once you understand the bigger logic of the system you're in, you can make intelligent and workable changes to get the result you want.

Chapter 7: Working with Goals and Visions

Let Vison Power Your Decision

Let's continue a little further with the idea of decisiveness. There are plenty of reasons that people do things, but not all reasons are created equal. If you act out of peer pressure, the expectations of others, or guilt, you may get some things done, but your motivation won't last. It's far better to tap into those things that truly and genuinely fire you up and inspire you on the deepest level. It's this inspiration that will power you through the challenges and obstacles you're bound to encounter on your path.

Creating a personal vision statement may sound kind of cheesy, but it's actually a powerful way to start fueling your goals at the source. Understanding your real values and core principles give you courage to make the difficult decision to improve your life, and it keeps you going when times are tough. If you have a sense of purpose, you will without doubt experience greater and more lasting reserves of self-discipline and motivation than if you had only a superficial grasp on your actions.

A personal vision statement gives you direction and focus. It provides the criteria against which you can compare all your actions and decisions. The values in it are your guiding light. If you make a decision inspired by these principles, it's likely to be a great decision that actively brings you closer to the life you want to live. Let your vision power your decision!

Think of your vision statement as a chance to really explore everything you could be, and everything you aspire to be. A vision statement is like a set of life rules or a manifesto that tells you how you should act—how you could act—*from your highest principles*, and not from fear or laziness or obligation. If you were filled with self-doubt and conflicting desires, and if you were disorganized or unclear on what you were doing, you'd balk at the first challenge and find yourself struggled to be disciplined. But when you act from your vision, it's like you're plugged into the most potent energy source there is—purpose.

How to Use This in Your Life Immediately

Finding your purpose is not a superficial task you do in twenty minutes. In fact, these questions are so big they'll take your entire life to figure out. Nevertheless, here are some thoughts to help guide you—and remember, it's *your* inner conscience that is ultimately what you need to be checking in with:

In the broadest sense, what is your purpose, not just regarding your current goals, but your life in general? To learn? To love? To build a family? To go on an adventure and have fun? To create?

If nobody else's opinion mattered, and money was no object, what would you focus on? Why?

What things do you pour your heart and soul into purely for its own sake?

What have you been drawn to even as a child?

If you could write down ten "life rules" that you lived by forever, what would they be?

Now, as you're exploring these things, get more specific—what actions, thoughts, beliefs, and attitudes align with this greater purpose? Picture your ideal person or a perfect version of yourself. What do they do every day? How do they speak and what people are they surrounded with?

The next part is difficult—ask yourself how your current life compares to this vision. Where are actively behaving against your own core values? What actions could you take (today and in the long term) that would align you more closely with what really matters?

The thing is, self-discipline and motivation should be *in service of* something. Why waste energy and willpower forcing yourself to do things that are ultimately not your highest calling? Reserve your energy, your hope, and your blood sweat and tears for the things that you know deep down will give your life a sense of meaning.

Be Decisive and Committed
Who doesn't want better self-discipline? The truth is, however, that self-discipline is more of a *how* than a *what*. We get more self-discipline in life not because we have made the disciplined life our goal, but rather that we have committed to another goal that we have set our sights on. A goal that inspires us to be better, that speaks to our values, and that fires up our motivation to create the things we most care about. Self-discipline is then the manner in which we embark on reaching that goal.

Sometimes, if you find yourself lacking discipline, it may not be a question of laziness or poor time management or unclear goals. Rather, you may have skipped over the *decision* to actually do your tasks, day after day, in order to reach your goal. Yes, at some point, you need to make the clear decision about what you're going to do and commit to it. All the planning and strategizing in the world mean nothing until you sit with yourself and say, "Okay. This is happening now. I've made a decision."

This is not a step to skip. Being decisive is about becoming a better decision-maker. When you make a decision, you are gathering information, narrowing it down, weighing up the pros and cons, and *making an agreement with yourself* that things are going to be different now. We ordinarily think of making decisions as a way to choose between various options offered, or resolve a tricky situation as best we can. But decisiveness goes deeper than that—it is also the act of us saying to ourselves that a threshold has been crossed, and from now on it is we who are in charge, and we are now steering the ship of where our life goes.

Some people call this commitment, and it is. If we identify our goal and the path to get there, committing to it means we have decided how we will act, no matter what temptations arise or how difficult it is. Have you ever met a person who, for example, quit smoking cold turkey, saying, "I just decided I wasn't going to do it anymore, and so I didn't"? It's because they decided, they committed, and that was that.

Being more decisive in life means having a good reputation with yourself and trusting your own word. When you follow through on your commitments, you trust and respect yourself more, and realize that self-discipline is more for those who are wavering in their decision. You are automatically more focused because you simply don't pay attention to other options, i.e., all those choices that take you away from your path.

If you lack decisiveness, it will show up as overanalyzing, getting stuck in "research" and not taking action, second-guessing yourself, having poor boundaries, succumbing to temptation, people-pleasing, perfectionism, and feeling like you're not totally convinced about the value of your goal in the first place. This is a sign that you need to stop, look at what you're doing and refresh both your decision and your commitment.

How to Use This in Your Life Immediately

Simply making a decision doesn't mean you're making a good one. You'll feel more conviction in your dedication if the decision actually makes sense for you.

Step 1: Reconsider your goal. Is it clear? Appropriate? Something you actually want? Take your time to visualize it and find your passion for it again.

Step 2: Reconnect with reasons . . . and consequences. Remind yourself of why you're trying to achieve your goal and also what you're trying to avoid. Remind yourself of the bad outcomes of following other paths, like procrastinating and giving up.

Step 3: Realize that nobody makes the decision but you—nobody else can! You are solely responsible for your own happiness and success. Clear away everyone else's opinions or expectations and enjoy your own agency.

Step 4: Now, choose. Tell yourself that this is how you will act because you have set your mind and it's what you want. Simple but powerful.

Step 5: Adjust as you go. Yes, you can have a concrete, iron will. But that doesn't mean you aren't constantly scanning for opportunities to go for an even better decision in future.

Goals: Identify Them and Write Them Down

A goal without a concrete plan of action is just a dream! In other words, it's never going to happen. Goal setting is the conscious and deliberate process of identifying the outcome you want to achieve, so that you can make appropriate plans for arriving at that objective. So, there are two parts: the goal, and the plan to get there. The destination and the map. To succeed you need to know where you're going, but you also need to know how you're going to get there.

Setting appropriate goals takes intelligence and self-discipline, but having goals in place is also something that inspires self-discipline, since it keeps us focused and on the path. When you are specific, plan carefully, and organize yourself, you have a greater chance of actually turning that abstract goal into concrete reality for yourself.

People often fail to make goals because it seems kind of obvious. They think they already know in sufficient detail what they want, so they dive in with the plan. Or, they think that dwelling on the outcome is enough, and that the plan to get there will work itself out somehow. This is just a recipe for staying exactly how you have always been.

You've probably already heard of SMART goals, but this is not the only way to structure your goal-setting strategy. Good goals tend to share a few common characteristics:

- They're actionable (remember, action is the bridge between potential and actual)
- They're clearly defined (vagueness = lack of commitment)
- They're meaningful to you (there's a big *why* behind them)
- They're set on a fixed timeline with small actionable steps on the way
- They're flexible and can be adjusted as you go
- They're visible and current to keep you accountable (usually, that means written down)

As long as your goal-setting approach includes these elements, you're off to a good start.

How to use this in your life immediately

A great goal-setting tool is called FAST.

According to this model, goals should be Frequently discussed. This means you have the chance to appraise progress and make minor course corrections as you go. Creating a goal is one thing, but it needs to be kept alive. Keep re-visiting it and asking if you're on track and how to accommodate unexpected changes. Do you need to tighten up your focus or work in some feedback?

Goals should also be **A**mbitious. You're not plodding along, but striving to be the best you can be. Even if you achieve a milestone, ask if you can do more, and how. Can you adjust your goal by aiming higher? Sometimes, ambition takes the form of creativity—see if you can find truly innovative ways to maximize what you're working with.

Goals should be **S**pecific. This is perhaps the most important characteristic from the better-known SMART goal method. You want to be as clear and detailed as possible. Use vivid visualization to be ultra-clear and concise with what you're trying to achieve.

Finally, goals should be **T**ransparent. This applies more to a team context, but it basically refers to full understanding of the role you play as a stakeholder in the outcome. You need to know what your tasks are and exactly how they contribute to the final goal. It's about clearly and appropriately mapping out the relationship between the tasks you're doing and the goal—they need to be as aligned as possible.

The benefit of this approach is that you focus more on ambition and flexibility, which may ultimately make you feel more inspired and more able to grow with your goals rather than be beholden to them. As you make your goal, run it through the FAST acronym and see if you've ticked all the boxes.

When in Doubt, Write it Out
When you get clear with yourself and home in on what you want to do, and commit to doing it, that's all that's strictly needed. However, we've seen that it's also very useful to externalize this conscious decision by writing it down or making your dedication to your goal visible to you at all times. The idea is pretty straightforward—those things that we

write down and read in black and white appeal to our unconscious mind as *more real* somehow. When we keep affirmations, goals, or a progress chart somewhere visible, we're constantly reminded of the path we're on, and stay aware of our mission.

But the power of writing goes beyond this. We can use the written word as a space to help us fine-tune our self-discipline and include it in our daily routine. When in doubt, write it out. Get out a notebook and pen, slow down, and put your thoughts in writing. This helps you focus, get organized, and look for emerging themes and patterns. What's more, when you have a written record of what you've already done, this gives you perspective, and reminds you of all the obstacles you've already overcome. It allows you to get a bigger picture on the daily trials and tribulations and see the broader, positive progression you're making—i.e., don't give up!

Putting your thoughts down helps you clarify what they actually are, and this helps with your decision-making processes, your creativity and your ability to analyze your own thinking. How does this relate to willpower? As you've noticed, we refer again and again to the power of awareness and intention. Think of the blank page as a workspace where you can play out your intentions, and practice becoming more aware not only of what's going on now, but of what's happened in the past, and how you might like to shape the future. This cannot help but sharpen your self-discipline and focus. In fact, many people look to their journals and diaries as a kind of "self-therapy"— whenever they're wavering in their resolve, they stop, get out the notebook, and pick through their thoughts and feelings until they have clarity and insight again.

How to Use This in Your Life Immediately

The great thing about a writing habit is that you can make it what you want it to be. You can have journals of all kinds, diaries, a simple system of notes and memos, or indulge your creative side by writing stories or poetry. You could mix everything up and have a book where you keep reflections, affirmations, goals and daily to-do lists, and any sudden ideas that pop up and which you want to capture before you forget them.

First things first: when you sit down to write, abandon the idea of what you *should* be doing. Really, it's up to you. But here are some ideas to get you started:

- Take a snapshot of where your attention is currently going by doing a kind of "brain dump"—put everything in your mind down on paper, and then without judgment, have a look and sift through it. This can help you process emotions.
- Make lists. Make a gratitude list, or a list of all the things you're dreaming big about. List out everything that's bothering you. Do the Stoic exercise from earlier in the book. Or simply write down a list of anxious ruminations that you then burn or tear up and say, "I'm done worrying about you now."
- Gather inspiring quotes, affirmations, poems, or mottos that

help focus your motivation and remind you why you're doing what you're doing. Some people like to put these at the top of every page so they can constantly see them.

Get Comfortable with Uncomfortable

The story sometimes goes like this: you get a big idea for a goal you'd like to achieve, you make a plan, get buzzed about it, and start on your path. Then, you encounter something awful or boring or confusing or something way, way harder than you expected it to be. You get scared. You get "tired." You slink away, forgetting your previous sense of motivation and energy. What happened?

To a large degree, your success in life is not defined by the grandiosity and beauty of your visions for yourself. Rather, it comes down to how willing you are to honestly and bravely face all those other things-- delay, failure, confusion, difficulty, pain, embarrassment, disappointment. Too often we plan our path toward our goal with the unconscious expectation that nothing will go wrong. When it does (inevitably) go wrong, we're unprepared and disillusioned by it.

The truth is that cultivating self-discipline to achieve our goals is really about seeking change. And if we want life to change, we have to risk leaving behind the old and familiar, and getting comfortable with the new and unfamiliar. This is not optional—change *is* uncomfortable. An invaluable asset to cultivate for yourself is a positive and healthy relationship to change, uncertainty, and discomfort. Most people never even realize that they have a choice in how they can approach and work with "negative emotions"!

This has ramifications for self-discipline. If you are unwilling to be uncomfortable, you run away when things get tough, and you play safe and refuse to take risks. You may steer clear of difficult conversations at home and at work. Afraid of conflict, you may fail to challenge yourself or others, to greater performance and a better life. When you stay small, you are also damaging your self-respect and self-confidence, never giving yourself the chance to demonstrate that you can rise above and do better, or the satisfaction of achievement.

But if you expect, understand and don't fear change and discomfort, you don't allow it to control you. You play outside your comfort zone, overcome obstacles, and are receptive to learning new things. A great attitude to have is to simply never expect comfort or certainty—think of both of these things as close to *death*, while change, risk, novelty, and unpredictability are closer to *life*.

How to Use This in Your Life Immediately

The next time something bad, unexpected, scary or uncomfortable happens, just pause a moment. Inwardly thank life for sending you a lovely lesson and a challenge through which you can improve and learn. Take a moment to remind yourself of one important fact: change is a part of life, but you always possess the ability to navigate any change through your own personal power and commitment.

Thus, instead of seeing what didn't happen for you, ask what else could happen. Instead of feeling sad that you failed, become curious about what lessons are still waiting to be learned. Instead of fearing some new and strange situation, embrace it with curiosity and the creativity it takes to launch out and try something different. It's all a matter of perspective. We don't need to make change or uncertainty the enemy. We can work with them.

You can always choose to become aware and orient yourself in the present moment, right now. What's going on? How do you feel? Why? Are you in real danger or just perceived danger? What are the stories you're telling about this situation?

If you fail, embrace it. It's as good a teacher as success. Acknowledge how you feel, learn what you can, make any changes that are in your scope of agency, then take action. Trust deep down that success or failure says nothing about your worth as a person. Failure, then, is just data, and what matters is what you do with that precious information.

Sometimes people fear change because they don't believe they have what it takes to survive it. This is why one more thing you can do to get comfortable with discomfort is to remind yourself that you are, in fact, capable. Remember precious success and remind yourself of all those times you were uncomfortable before, but how it all worked out in the end. If you can, remind yourself also of how staying in your comfort zone ultimately wasn't as great as it seemed at the time—perhaps you have regrets about all those times you could have pushed yourself but didn't.

You have the power to shape outcomes. You have the ability to choose your mindset, and you can take actions that align with your values—there is great confidence in knowing that you always have this right, even when things seem hard or boring or scary or strange.

Takeaways:

- The most powerful way to energize your decisions and be self-disciplined is to connect to your greater life visions, and what your ultimate purpose is. Make decisions from your vision. When you are powered by your own personal vision statement, you act from principle and are far more likely to be motivated and stay the course.
- The tips we've discussed will help foster more self-discipline, but at some point, you will need to make the clear decision and commitment toward achieving your dreams. Think about your goal and the reasons for having that goal, and then

take responsibility for choosing that and committing to the path. Nobody can commit on your behalf—it is your decision alone.

- Good goal-setting goes beyond making SMART goals. Try the alternative FAST goals: make them frequently discussed and reworked, ambitious (why not go for gold?), specific, and transparent, i.e., make sure you understand how every action you take connects to the goal at the end. Goals should be flexible and inspiring. Don't be afraid to change things up or push yourself to do more once you've reached a milestone.
- Any growth takes courage to weather the discomfort of change. Adopt a mindset where you expect, welcome, and understand discomfort, and don't fear uncertainty. Don't allow negative emotions, setbacks, confusion, failure, or adversity to deter you from your mission. Getting comfortable with the uncomfortable also means reminding yourself that you are capable and able to access your own power and choice to make good decisions, no matter what happens.

Summary Guide

CHAPTER 1: GETTING STARTED

- When cultivating the self-discipline needed to achieve your goals, it matters how you start. Forego quantum leaps and overnight successes and instead "think small" by breaking your big goal down into manageable, sustainable baby steps. What matters most is habit and consistency.
- You have more chance of achieving your goal if you make a conscious "fresh start," i.e., begin on New Year's Day, your birthday, or the first day of the week, Monday. Deliberately and consciously mark the occasion and make it memorable, telling yourself that the past is forgiven and forgotten, and you are turning over a new leaf.

- Make a promise to yourself that even though you may occasionally have setbacks, you will never skip your task for two days in a row. One day is understandable, but two days makes a habit. If you slip up, go into learning mode and ask why so you can ensure you don't do the same the following day.
- Choose a goal, set a timeframe, and then choose some appropriate metrics to track and monitor your progression. Keep this visible and concrete, to inspire you, give you a sense of focus and accomplishment, and help you troubleshoot and pre-empt problems.
- Finally, use the power of visualization to train your brain in the right direction. Draw on all five senses to imagine the desired outcome or the process toward that outcome—or both. What matters is that you do it regularly and really delve into the *feelings* associated with what you're trying to create.

CHAPTER 2: FOCUS ON HABITS

- To become more disciplined, focus on your bad habits and work not to eliminate them but replace them with better ones. Observe your current habits, understand the purpose they serve, their triggers and their results, and take action to rework them in your favor. With good habits in place, you need *less* self-discipline, not more.
- It sounds basic, but you cannot cultivate self-discipline without the foundation of a healthy lifestyle. You can fuel your willpower by considering how to fuel your body first. There are many different diet philosophies, and they all work, but one thing consistently shown to improve self-control is to maintain stable blood sugar levels.
- Regular exercise will boost your self-esteem, fill your body with endorphins, keep you fit and strong, and help you exercise your resolve as you exercise your muscles. Remember: how you do anything is how you do everything. Exercise not only your body but your mind.
- If you don't have one already, establish a rock-solid morning routine that gets you started on the right foot. Each person

has their own unique biorhythms, but most of us benefit from having regular sleep and wake times and healthy sleep habits.
- Give yourself less work to do by having a weekly schedule, which is built around your priorities. Cluster less important tasks together and build in some wiggle room and time to appraise and adjust.
- Make sure you are scheduling in ample time to rest and recuperate, as well as time to acknowledge your progress and reward yourself. This is crucial for your ongoing success!

CHAPTER 3: GET RIGHT IN YOUR BODY, MIND AND SOUL

- Getting right in body, mind, and soul means adopting the attitudes and mindsets that make a self-disciplined life possible. Firstly, make a plan to reduce, remove, and avoid temptations. If you are proactive and pre-empt them, they have less impact on your life.
- One of the biggest and most damaging myths is that we can only take action

when the time is right or when we feel like it. The truth is that we can act even if we don't have the motivation! Just start, and you'll find that it's the other way around: taking action inspires you.
- Don't beat yourself up—nobody every improved from a position of judgment and self-hate. Have compassion for yourself, be kind, forgive slip-ups, and keep focusing on the positives. You do not need to make yourself feel bad in order to improve.
- We all have moods that change and shift, but we also possess the ability to choose how we respond. We can allow ourselves to feel what we feel without letting moods disrupt our goals or commitment. Notice your moods as moods and choose not to react to them. Act instead from your rational, conscious mind.
- Willpower is a limited resource that can get depleted on the many tiny stressors and tensions of daily life. Lower your overall life stress and you free up more mental bandwidth to spend on what's really important. Stress management should be a regular habit and not

reserved for when you're already struggling.
- Finally, think of glucose as the physical analogue of willpower. Sip something sweet to replenish glucose (which your brain runs on) and you improve your self-control—just make sure you're not overindulging in unhealthy sweet things.

CHAPTER 4: THE ATTITUDE OF SUCCESS

- Your success is determined by your attitude. Get real and honest with yourself and remove those things in life that seem like they're making you productive but are actually just wasting your time. Keep asking, "Does this move me forward?"
- Use positive peer pressure to keep you accountable to your commitments. Rope in friends to witness your achievements, support you, and inspire you when you're having trouble.
- Have a healthy attitude toward control—though there are things in life we never have control over, we are

always in charge of our own reactions and actions. Try the Stoic exercise to help you identify what you can change, what you can't, and practice the wisdom it takes to know the difference.
- Self-disciplined people know that their success in life is their own responsibility, and they own it. They don't blame others, complain, or wait for permission. They embrace the freedom of responsibility.
- A regular gratitude practice keeps you in a positive frame of mind, makes you more resilient, more creative, and better able to control yourself. Find things to be thankful for every single day, and fill yourself up with good feelings that make self-discipline easier.
- Finally, if you believe you can do it, you can. Self-belief is a powerful predictor of success, so have a little faith in yourself!

CHAPTER 5: STAY MINDFUL

- Being mindful and meditating are not just ways to reduce stress and improve wellbeing; they're techniques to strengthen self-awareness, lower reactivity and improve self-discipline. When you meditate, you activate the parts of your brain responsible for self-control, strengthening those neural connections.
- Meditation is not just a discrete activity but a way of life. Find ways to become aware throughout the day and use these feelings of calm control and mindfulness to reconnect to your self-discipline. Pause, become aware of what's going on inside you and outside you in your environment, and notice your thoughts and feelings without judgment or interpretation.
- A major stumbling block for those wanting to develop better self-discipline and improve their lives as letting their ego get in the way. The ego is a mask; it's not the real you. Regularly remind yourself of the process, not the outcome and be okay with being a beginner or being wrong. Stop playing a role and encounter the moment as it is—no comparisons, appraisals, or judgments.

- On your self-discipline journey, you'll encounter pain, which is inevitable. But suffering (i.e., the way we react to pain) is avoidable. Blame, personal narratives, regret, self-hate, doubt, anxiety etc. are all optional reactions. Try not to add "second darts" when life deals you a bad hand. With awareness and calm, compassionate acceptance, we can allow both pain and suffering to pass.
- Knowledge is power, and self-knowledge is self-power. If you know your strengths and weaknesses, you can consciously work around your blind spots while maximizing on your good attributes. Don't see your flaws as shortcomings, but instead learn what you can from them and focus on the good.

CHAPTER 6: GET ORGANIZED WITH YOUR TIME

- Willpower is a limited resource but so is time. Self-discipline requires conscious control over how we spend our time. Follow Stephen Covey's advice and "put the big rocks first"—the less important

tasks of life can be squeezed in later. Start the day with your priorities.
- Not everyone will follow the same sleep/wakefulness cycles; it's up to you to understand your own rhythms and work with them. Identify your peak energy periods and schedule your most important or demanding tasks for this time. You need less self-discipline if you're working with your natural motivational flow.
- A great way to break out of inaction or overcome strong derailing emotions is to count down from ten and then just force yourself to act. Anxiety can be tackled by becoming aware of the present moment on all five senses. Anger can be managed by hitting the pause button, breathing deeply, and having a time out.
- Procrastination can be a sign that your organization, goals or mindset are not where they should be, but all of us procrastinate out of laziness from time to time. Fix the problem by restoring momentum as soon as you can. Get started with just the tiniest task first or promise yourself you'll do just five minutes. If your procrastination comes

from deeper issues, you need to tackle these first.
- A to-do list can help focus you, but if you're a chronic over-doer, a don't-do list may be more appropriate. Look at every item on your list and ask whether it is urgent and important. Tasks that are neither can be ignored or delegated, tasks that are both should be prioritized.
- Finally, become adept at noticing your own behavioral patterns. Be mindful, honest and proactive in recognizing where you're repeating the same patterns over and over. Once you understand the bigger logic of the system you're in, you can make intelligent and workable changes to get the result you want.

CHAPTER 7: WORKING WITH GOALS AND VISIONS

- The most powerful way to energize your decisions and be self-disciplined is to connect to your greater life visions, and what your ultimate purpose is. Make decisions from your vision. When you

are powered by your own personal vision statement, you act from principle and are far more likely to be motivated and stay the course.
- The tips we've discussed will help foster more self-discipline, but at some point, you will need to make the clear decision and commitment toward achieving your dreams. Think about your goal and the reasons for having that goal, and then take responsibility for choosing that and committing to the path. Nobody can commit on your behalf—it is your decision alone.
- Good goal-setting goes beyond making SMART goals. Try the alternative FAST goals: make them frequently discussed and reworked, ambitious (why not go for gold?), specific, and transparent, i.e., make sure you understand how every action you take connects to the goal at the end. Goals should be flexible and inspiring. Don't be afraid to change things up or push yourself to do more once you've reached a milestone.
- Any growth takes courage to weather the discomfort of change. Adopt a mindset where you expect, welcome, and understand discomfort, and don't

fear uncertainty. Don't allow negative emotions, setbacks, confusion, failure, or adversity to deter you from your mission. Getting comfortable with the uncomfortable also means reminding yourself that you are capable and able to access your own power and choice to make good decisions, no matter what happens.

www.ingramcontent.com/pod-product-compliance
Lightning Source LLC
Chambersburg PA
CBHW011130070526
44583CB00023B/2972